The Birth of the Patient

The Birth of the Patient

Multiple Entities of Newborns in Russian Neonatal Care

Anastasia Novkunskaya, Artemiy Minakov and Anna Klepikova

LEXINGTON BOOKS
Lanham • Boulder • New York • London

Lexington Books
Bloomsbury Publishing Inc, 1385 Broadway, New York, NY 10018, USA
Bloomsbury Publishing Plc, 50 Bedford Square, London, WC1B 3DP, UK
Bloomsbury Publishing Ireland, 29 Earlsfort Terrace, Dublin 2, D02 AY28, Ireland
www.rowman.com

British Library Cataloguing in Publication Information Available

Library of Congress Cataloging-in-Publication Data Available

ISBN 9781666937404 (cloth : alk. paper) | ISBN 9781666937411 (ebook)

For product safety related questions contact productsafety@bloomsbury.com.

Contents

Acknowledgements vii

Introduction ix

List of Abbreviations xv

1 The Big Case of Micropaediatrics: The Institutionalisation of Neonatal Care 1

2 In Searching for the Point of View 25

3 Nothing Personal 43

4 Emotional Dimension of Neonatal Care 65

5 Managerial, Economic and Political Entities of a Newborn 129

Conclusion 189

Appendix 1: Guide for Expert and Biographical Interviews with Medical Professionals Involved in the Institutionalization of Neonatology Since the Late 1970s 199

Appendix 2: Guide for a Focus Group with Physicians and Nurses in the Neonatology Service 201

Appendix 3: List of Informants and Description of Interviews 205

Appendix 4: List of Observations 209

Appendix 5: List and Description of Focus Groups 213

Appendix 6: List of Archival Documents 217

References 219

Index 231

About the Authors 235

Acknowledgements

This book would be impossible without so many people – our parents, partners, children and other loved ones who supported us during the fieldwork and manuscript writing process. However, we will not list our thanks individually but would like to acknowledge the participation, help and advice of those colleagues who made it possible for us to come together as a team and realise the whole project.

First of all, we would like to thank Ekaterina Borozdina, without whose outstanding organisational, communicative and human qualities we simply would not have met each other. It was she who assembled and directed the programme on Social Research in Health and Medicine at the European University at St. Petersburg, to which Artemy enrolled, and the empirical field of observation of the neonatology service began. We also thank all the faculty of this programme, our colleagues and the administrative staff of the European University who discussed the first results of the work and helped us with educational, research and bureaucratic tasks over the years. Particularly, we would like to acknowledge the contribution of Ilya Utekhin, who reviewed Artemy's graduate work and provided inspiration to get the results published and helped us with proofreading and indexation. We would also like to thank the administrators of the Interdisciplinary Institute for Health Research, Polina Tazenkova and Maria Okuneva, who helped us with all the necessary paperwork, documents, coordination of data transcriptions and translation of some parts of the text. We thank those people who helped us with the translation of the text and transcription of interviews and focus group data. We also thank the corporate donor of the Associated Professorship on Qualitative Health Research for financial support of the data transcriptions and manuscript translation.

We are grateful to all of our colleagues who provided us with emotional support, as well as valuable critical comments and analytical advice in the process of working on the research and the text. In particular, Maria Pirogovskaia and Ekaterina Khonineva, who provided advice for the chapter on emotions, Daria Litvina, with whom we discussed some issues at the intersection of our and her empirical fields, those colleagues who gave us feedback at conferences where we presented the intermediate results of our work: Natalia Mitsyuk, Anna Belova, Olga Simonova and Kristin Kay Barker in particular.

This book would also not have been possible without the initiative and continued support of the editors of Lexington Books. We thank Ryan Dradzynski, Emma Ebert, Courtney Morales and Jasper Mislak for their patience, answering all our questions and providing guidance and support throughout the entire manuscript. We also thank the anonymous reviewer of our manuscript for his or her positive feedback and very helpful and relevant recommendations for revisions. We warmly thank our colleagues Vladislav Gorodetskiy and Andrey Tolokonnikov, who created photos during their work and agreed to provide them for the book cover.

We cannot name our research participants, in order to provide their anonymity; however, we would like to express our deepest gratitude to all of them – in particular, we are grateful to the senior Resuscitation and Advisory Centre colleagues who not only taught the profession but also allowed us to touch the past. In addition, we acknowledge the invaluable assistance provided by Viktoria Kuznetsova and Julia Agapova, who helped us recruit nurses working in maternity hospitals for our focus groups. We would also like to thank all the small patients who we met during the research and who, in fact, made the research possible, and we wish them good luck in all their trajectories.

Introduction

Some classical social theories (see, for example, Parsons 1951b) and the 'medical gaze' (health practitioners and systems of healthcare) often consider a patient as a consistent category and phenomenon. However, of late different studies problematise this idea by noting that patients have different social characteristics and cultural backgrounds and, depending on their health condition and the disease afflicting them, they would follow different trajectories within medical institutions and acquire different experiences (Roth 1972; Lorber 1975; Najman et al. 1982; Kirmayer and Robbins 1996; Nápoles-Springer et. al. 2005; Kleinman 2020; Litvina 2022). Our book contributes to this long-lasting discussion and examines a (newborn) patient from different perspectives within the same medical context, comprising the neonatal resuscitation service within one region of Russia. Such a design and conceptual framework, on the one hand, allows us to uncover the universal mechanisms for constructing the social position of a patient depending on the institutional settings framing it. On the other, it enables us to demonstrate in detail that the same patient within the same institutional context appears in practice in many different entities.

The study was conducted in one of the Russian regions, where intensive care for newborns in most cases is mediated by the resuscitation and advisory centre (RAC). This department is engaged in the registration, remote monitoring, counselling and transportation of newborns born in maternity facilities who require resuscitation or intensive care. The centre works with both maternity and children's hospitals, providing newborn patients with access to high-tech and surgical care. All facilities and departments involved in neonatal resuscitation care provision can be divided into three sectors: obstetrics (maternity hospitals and departments), resuscitation and advisory centre, and the sector of children's hospitals. The obstetrics sector is represented by maternity hospitals and obstetric departments in multidisciplinary hospitals, which provide medical care to both women and newborn children. The sector of paediatric hospitals, as a rule, is represented by multidisciplinary clinics, mainly restoring children's health with subsequent discharge or transferring to rehabilitation departments. Children are the only kind of patients receiving care in this sector. The resuscitation and advisory centre, often referred to as RAC, is an intermediate transit sector that includes both inpatient and ambulance medical care. The practices that are carried out in this sector are associated with short-term therapeutic procedures and include intensive communication with representatives of other sectors.

In a number of conditions and circumstances, the patient's status turns out to be almost the only thing that sets the order of social interactions, and his or her social characteristics, on the contrary, are linked to the already existing medicalised position. This research focuses on such interactions between medical professionals and patients, in which the role of a patient chronologically and symbolically is primary, preceding other social roles. The title of the book *The Birth of the Patient* refers both to the object and subject of the research. Firstly, the focus is on data collected in the context of neonatal care, that is, care for newborns and, therefore, the profile of medicine that is directly related to the moment of birth. Secondly, we propose to turn to the analysis of how the image of a patient and his or her social statuses are constructed in such a medicalised context.

We are certainly not the first scholars to address the empirical field of resuscitation and to explore how different social characteristics of a patient can influence their interactions with medical institutions, and how many different social perspectives constitute the social order of this field (see, for example, Anspach 1993; Wamsiedel 2023). A key contribution of our research within this discussion is that we do not focus on the moral dimension of the decision to resuscitate or not resuscitate patients and how their triage is organised and practised. The focus of our research is the complex of different dimensions of professional work in neonatal resuscitation, including but not limited to the moral dimensions of life-and-death decisions. The book addresses the multiplicity of social perspectives and contexts, which frame the position and the entities of a newborn patient within the medical community and the medical institutional settings. We aim to show that patients with similar social characteristics and within similar organisational contexts actually appear in different 'essences' or 'entities': physical, social, economic and even political. At the same time, dealing with a patient 'without personal biography' (such as a newborn, especially born prematurely) and in some cases 'without future' (as some of them have very high risks of adverse outcomes), the study uncovers the universal mechanisms of constructing the medical position of a patient, depending on the institutional settings in which he or she occurs. The development of our narrative successively and in detail tells the story of *The Birth of the Patient.*

Chapter 1, 'The Big Case of Micropaediatrics: The Institutionalisation of Neonatal Care', introduces the key research question, which is the multiplicity of the social and cultural statuses of a newborn patient, shaped and framed by the historical, political, cultural, economic and medical contexts. The narrative in this chapter successively reveals the background of neonatal care in Russia, its history, organisational arrangement, and the way of governance and regulation. First, we consider how in the early 1980s neonatal care was provided without a specific organisational frame, but based only on the initiative of particular specialists, and how gradually it became institutionalised. We examine in detail how technological innovations have changed the way neonatal care is provided and organised.

Secondly, in this chapter, we show how the field of neonatology is currently structured based on the evidence from Saint-Petersburg: which organisations and medical professionals provide such care, how medical specialists receive the necessary education, training and practice, and how both organisations and professionals coordinate with each other to provide neonatal care. Third, we focus on the way this field is regulated: what laws govern it, how control over neonatal care is structured and implemented, and how broader welfare and pronatalist policies affect the work of both neonatal care providers and the experiences of patients and their families.

Chapter 2, 'In Searching for the Point of View', consists of the description of the research design, methods applied to collect and analyse the data and reflections on the ethical and methodological collisions, arising with the participatory observation on the one hand and an interdisciplinary research team on the other.

The interdisciplinary approach to the field under study deserves special attention. As we co-authors have professionalised in different disciplines (sociology, anthropology and medicine), personally and professionally we view and construct 'patients' differently, as well as the arrangement of healthcare and the role of healthcare professionals involved in its provision. This interdisciplinarity in our standpoints, research positions, methods applied and interpretations of the data considerably shapes our ethnography and becomes a particular point of reflection. The major uniqueness here consists of the professional background and research position of one of the co-authors, who works as a neonatologist-resuscitator and has collected most of the empirical data. The unique experience of Artemiy, who is both the researcher and research participant, allows him not only to provide original ethnographic data but also to contribute to the methodological and ethical discussion on the advantages and limits of participatory observation.

Our key point is that research methods are not just instruments for collecting and analysing empirical data but a self-sufficient focus of research reflection. Thus, the sections of the chapter uncover the multiple ethical dilemmas and methodological challenges emerging during the ethnographic work, featured by the extremely sensitive research field, participatory observation and the interdisciplinary approach of the research team. The particular focus of reflection is on the combination of different professional and disciplinary perspectives regarding the same situations, as well as on the way different professional roles can be switched in case of providing emergency and intensive care.

In chapter 3, 'Nothing Personal', we show that medicalisation need not be seen solely in terms of the biomedical gaze dominance and its dehumanising nature regarding newborns in a number of social situations. We argue that medicalisation might rather be viewed as a spectrum of both social contexts and the attitudes of the medical personnel towards their patients. First, we show that depending on the severity of a patient's condition and the particular institutional settings the patient is placed in, the level of medicalisation may vary a lot. Second, analysing the empirical data, we view the process of medicalisation through the social labels used by healthcare practitioners in regard to newborns. We show that the objectification of patients is not aimed at their dehumanisation. Rather, it serves as an instrument of communication between different professionals involved in the process of medical care in a particular case. Finally, we demonstrate that despite the fact that certain stages of providing medical help to newborns are extremely medicalised, such patients are endued with social statuses and characteristics, which, together with biomedical properties, may have influence upon their trajectories.

Chapter 4, 'Emotional Dimension of Neonatal Care', deals with the construction of a newborn patient through emotional attitudes and focuses on the emotional work, broadly understood, done by the medical staff. The patient under study in our case is a newborn baby who has not passed through socialisation yet, including the socialisation into the cultural ways of expressing emotions. Apart from that, newborn patients are most often kept under sedation, so they are deprived of the opportunity to express emotional signals that might be interpreted as discomfort or pain. Despite these difficulties, as we show, interaction with such patients in institutional settings is very sensitive and fused with emotions. Here, we focus on how the newborn patients' feelings and emotional states are reflected in and constructed by the reactions, emotions and practices of people who interact with them.

In particular, we turn to the concept of the 'extended patient' and, applying it to our ethnographic materials, we demonstrate that parents and relatives become the representatives of the patient in communication with the medical staff, and they contribute to the creation of the baby as an emotional entity.

We also show that though emotional work is an essential part of medical professionalism, different medical professionals practice it differently. Thus, nurses afford themselves more emotional involvement in communication with newborns, while the task of the physicians is to remain neutral even in the most sensitive situations. However, as we discovered, this priority of neutrality does not mean that they are emotionally detached or have no sympathy for the patients and their families. Rather, they have to develop a variety of coping strategies that they instrumentalise in the most dramatic moments, including the patient's death.

Chapter 5, 'Managerial, Economic and Political Entities of a Newborn', tells the documentary and bureaucratic story of a newborn. The system of Russian healthcare, in general, is characterised by the perpetual transformation caused by post-socialist (and, in practice, neoliberal) reforms. Just like maternity care, neonatal care directly relates to the 'pronatalist' agenda, and, hence, it appears at the centre of the state's attention. It has undergone multiple reforms, causing changes in regulation, organisation and, as we argue, social communication in the field. In addition to this political course, recent historical events (the pandemic during 2020–2022, and the war since February 2022) appreciably affect both healthcare professionals' practices and patients' trajectories.

This chapter reveals how, in addition to the biomedical and social entities, a newborn appears in other ones, and how his or her trajectories are shaped by economic, political and bureaucratic processes. The particular focus is on the way a newborn patient appears as an abstract statistical unit that forms economic and reputational (symbolic) performance indicators for medical institutions. The chapter, on the one hand, describes the context of neonatal care as fairly strictly regulated. On the other hand, it depicts the stories that reveal the grey areas of this regulation – for instance, medical care provided to newborns without Russian citizenship. In particular, such cases reveal that even in such a medicalised and rigidly regulated context, the work of medical professionals and health managers can be aimed at constructing the cultural entity of a newborn and building a special trajectory for him or her beyond the institutionalised settings.

Analysing the empirical data, reflecting on the methodological aspects of our ethnographic study, and participating in the theoretical discussion on medicalisation, patients' agency and professionals' autonomy, we arrive at the key conclusions of the book. We, firstly, emphasise how political, biomedical, social, emotional and economic contexts and factors determine and constitute a newborn within the medical settings. Secondly, we contribute to the understanding of the medicalisation and the medical gaze – in particular, the way they shape the trajectory and the fate of a person, who by default appears immediately as a patient with limited agency and without having her or his own autonomous biography. We conclude that the ethnographic work of even a very specific local setting provides important insights into more universal principles of the work of medical institutions and health professionals.

Sensitivity of the field under study and the relatively closed nature of the medical institutions (especially those of resuscitation and intensive care) comprise an important feature of the book. Although we recognise some specificities of the context of study, we expect that some insights from the extremely medicalised neonatal care could be relevant to many others as well, as the issues of life and death, the medicalisation of childcare, professional autonomy and the institutional logics shaping neonatology in particular and healthcare in general are similar across different countries. And, finally, as we have conducted our fieldwork in 2019–2023, we claim that the changing institutional context under study, framed by post-socialist turbulence, the pandemic and the warfare is also quite unique. This feature is that in the process of collecting qualitative data that took place in very particular local settings, we can nevertheless observe the reflection of global historical changes that also shape the experience, trajectories and fate of a newborn patient.

List of Abbreviations

ALV – Artificial lung ventilation
FIF – Formalised information form
FMS – Federal Migration Service
ICU – Intensive Care Unit
IVF – In-vitro fertilisation
MHI – Mandatory Health Insurance
NICU – Neonatal Intensive Care Unit
PRC – People's Republic of China
RAC – Resuscitation and Advisory Centre (NRAC – Newborn Resuscitation and Advisory Centre, initial name of the same centre)
WHO – World Health Organisation

Chapter 1

The Big Case of Micropaediatrics

The Institutionalisation of Neonatal Care

Medicine as culture (Lupton 2012) is a field of scientific knowledge and a system of practices. Therefore, it influences the concept of 'normal' both within the medical community and in society as a whole. The resistance and attempts to maintain the status quo often accompany the adoption of new medical rules and regulations. Medical progress can result, whatever it might mean, in the expansion of the scope of biomedical knowledge and the transformation of society, which accepts or rejects this knowledge. This chapter shows how the concept of a newborn patient has changed in the medical world over a period of just over a hundred years, and how the system of medical care for newborns has been formed in one of the largest regions of Russia.

Although some patterns in the development of this system are considered to be common to other contexts, the purpose of this chapter is to show that even systems with strict and formalised regulation, a standardised organisational structure and a single concern have many local features and manifestations that refract general rules in different ways and create different practices. This work is trying to figure out what a newborn patient is like and deliberately focuses on the regional specifics of the research field – from the history of the issue to the modern model of care, remaining within the same region with its history, people, economic, social, cultural and bureaucratic features. The history of the institutionalisation of neonatal care in the region under study describes how technological and social innovations became key in this field, shaping its structural and cultural features at the present time rather than an 'objective' chronology of the key stages of its development.

THE FIRST INNOVATION IS HEAT

There is some information about newborns and their care in the centuries-old history of medicine. This chapter, however, starts from the period that marked a revolution in helping newborns and determined the further development of neonatology as a system of care not only for newborns but also for children born prematurely. This revolution drew a line between neonatology and paediatrics, just as earlier adult diseases were separated from childhood ones. In general, world history says children's hospitals as a separate type of institution appeared relatively late, that is, the very first children's hospital appeared in Paris in 1802 (C Jr, T. E. 1981); the second children's clinic in the world opened in the then capital of Russia, St. Petersburg 32 years later in 1834 (Radbill 1955). However, these institutions provided medical care to older children, while newborns were either observed by obstetricians or taken to orphanages and shelters, which were also planned and located separately from obstetric institutions and adult clinics.

The first month of a child's life, called a 'newborn period', is the adaptation to existence outside the mother's womb. If a child is born before 37 weeks[1] of gestation, this adaptation requires additional measures, that is, maintaining special external conditions, primarily a certain temperature and humidity. Those simple actions, which are aimed at creating an optimal physical environment, were the first and most significant steps that made it possible to nurse premature babies. However, in addition to the very opportunity to help these children, certain social and economic prerequisites should have been formed that would allow them to fight for every life. Undoubtedly, it meant spending significant resources on this and planning long-term measures. Historically, the value of a newborn's life, especially within the underprivileged social class, remained quite low (at least for a society) for a long time, mostly due to the common high infant death rate and high fertility rate.

In pre-revolutionary village culture, there was a traditional idea of the need to symbolically 'finish baking' or 'overbake' a child in an oven (Bayburin 1993, 53), which actually occupied a central place in family life. Villagers used the oven not only for cooking food but also for washing and warming children; they used it as a traditional treatment.

According to Leikin N. A., a member of the Saint-Petersburg Sanitary Commission, who raised the issue of care for premature babies in 1901, creating Russia's first asylum for premature babies in 1898: 'I was born . . . prematurely and for a long time was a frail child', who, in the absence of other opportunities, 'following the advice of various old women, was wrapped in tow (the fibre of flax prepared for spinning) and placed daily in a basket on the hearth of the Russian stove' (Leikin 1907).

It would be premature to call the stove the first analogue of the couveuse (incubator), but the very principle of using heat (temperature) as a therapeutic agent remains basic in modern intensive neonatology. The first analogues of modern couveuses appeared in the nineteenth century in Europe. As often happens in history, however, this invention appeared earlier than necessary and was untimely, given the demographic and social problems of that period. In 1889, the abovementioned Leikin proposed to the Saint-Petersburg Sanitary Commission to create and place French metal cabinets with glass ('maternité couveuse') and Viennese double-walled bathtubs in maternity hospitals as 'the first experiment'. Obstetricians rejected the initiative since they thought the placement of incubators in maternity hospitals could not significantly affect the nursing of premature babies. At that time, newborns were usually in shelters for no more than a week, which was not enough to provide proper neonatal care in preterm birth.

It is worth noting the importance of dialogue between obstetricians and future paediatricians from a historical perspective. Neonatology as a science belongs to obstetrics and paediatrics. For a long time, obstetricians were the only specialists who were engaged in the care of the newborn, and it was not until the early twentieth century, however, that paediatricians began to appear in obstetric institutions, which was the result of the heavy employment of obstetricians rather than special expertise: 'at large maternity hospitals, obstetricians have so much to do that a separate doctor should be appointed to monitor newborns . . . most likely a pediatrician' (Speransky 1914). The first paediatricians volunteered in obstetric institutions in large cities, and for a long time, they were not permanent staff of those institutions (Uspensky 1911, 131).

The first paediatricians appeared in obstetric institutions in 1906 (Novikov 2010). There was catastrophic infant mortality in the late nineteenth and early twentieth century in Russia. Contemporaries dubbed that time 'children's pestilence' because 268 out of 1,000 newborns died (Ivanov 1911, 35). According to some estimates, perinatal mortality in the region of research reached 100–150 ppm and one of the important factors was the 'fashion' for refusing breastfeeding [Ibid]. This fact made doctors pay more attention to paediatrics and contributed to the formation of this speciality. At the beginning of the twentieth century, issues of motherhood and childhood in the Russian Empire were resolved mainly through public initiatives. In 1904, the Union for the Fight against Infant Mortality was established, and later its branches were opened in other large cities (Ivanov, 1911). V. O. Hubert was one of the Union's members. He was leading the first Russian shelter for premature babies for eight years. The Union was collecting donations for the creation of consultations and milk stations 'Goutte de lait' ('Drop of Milk'), whose task was to promote breastfeeding, prepare formulas for newborns, including premature babies, and carry out educational work on child care. Until 1911, this consultation was financed by public funds and, subsequently, it was transferred under the control of the City Duma (Delektorsky 1910).

The decision to refuse to place incubators in maternity hospitals, made in 1889, can be considered the beginning of a large formation of the paediatric service as a separate system of care for infants (Shelkova 2022). Despite this refusal, the idea of caring for newborns did not disappear, and two years later a separate neonatal intensive care institution was opened to help premature babies. Before that time, surviving premature babies were brought to Orphanages, and mortality among children weighing less than 2,200g was about 30% (in 1986, 85 out of 292 children brought to the Orphanage died) (Central State Archive of Saint-Petersburg, F.210, Op.1, D. 32, L.3, cited after Zaerko 2017).

The first Russian shelter for premature babies was opened on 25 October 1901 (Zaerko 2017). It was designed for the simultaneous maintenance of ten premature babies during the first months of their lives. This shelter was located in a house owned by the city authorities. There already housed a smallpox vaccination institute, and in fact, it was a converted apartment with a large room for newborns, two rooms for nurses, a room for a paramedic, a dining room, a small laboratory 'for medical purpose', a kitchen and a small separate room that was a reception (Zaerko 2017). According to the existing information, that institution was quite successful. From 22 October 1901 to 1 January 1902, the Orphanage accepted 37 children, 16 of them weighing from 780 to 1,000g, 10 – from 1,010 to 1,500g, and 9 – from 1,540 to 2,000g, 2 – from 2,100 to 2,200g. Four newborns out of 37 died, 9 were in the institution on 1 January 1902 and 24 were discharged with significant weight gain. Later, that shelter moved to different locations and became one of the largest newborn care hospitals in the city.

By the end of the first decade of the twentieth century, paediatricians appeared in all major maternity hospitals in the capital and then in other large cities. In addition, separate baby care institutions were opened. They were not associated with obstetric hospitals, which indicated the final separation of paediatrics from obstetrics as a separate medical speciality (Gorelova and Shelkova 2022). A significant increase in the activity of public organisations and professional communities was observed in the Russian Empire at the end of the nineteenth century, including support for motherhood and childhood. Such efforts as providing consultations for low-income mothers who were breast-feeding, named 'Goutte du lait' and 'Union against child mortality', as well as voluntary paediatrician service in maternity shelters were the so-called grassroot initiatives at first, but subsequently they were institutionalised and became the basis for the future development of neonatal and paediatric care.

It is worth noting that similar processes took place outside of Russia, too. Initially, the idea of equipping maternity institutions in Europe and America with incubators was also rejected, which resulted in the appearance of alternative forms of medical institutions with elements of entertainment, for example, the famous fairs, which exhibited premature babies in incubators (Gras 2022). Such practices were reminiscent of the days of the anatomical theatres of Europe, where scientific and clinical tasks were carried out along with entertainment. On the other hand, they can be considered as an attempt to create the first open medical institutions. For example, Martin Arthur Couney charged 25 cents for the opportunity to see the struggling premature babies that he exhibited at the Coney Island Fair in Brooklyn. Thanks to these collections, he saved thousands of newborns. The first shelter for premature babies also meant public openness, considering it as part of educational work with the population:

> It is also important that the public was allowed free access to inspect the shelter, and for those, who wished, V. O. Gubert, the head of the shelter, gave explanations on the care of premature babies. (1901 Saint-Petersburg Executive Sanitary Commission Report, 1901, p. 75)

Modern neonatology as a medical discipline has a short but eventful history, in which not only technological innovations but also the active social position of the pioneers of this speciality have played an important role.

MEDICALISATION OF OBSTETRICS – NEW ORGANISATIONAL CHALLENGES

The birth of a child at home was considered the norm in Russia in the eighteenth and nineteenth centuries (Mitsyuk and Pushkareva 2021). Hospitals were built in metropolitan and large cities and were not popular. In 1913, the percentage of inpatient obstetric care was only 0.6% (Pavlova and Zelentsova 2020). Childbirth in those institutions was considered as the lot of women with low social status or women who found themselves in difficult life situations.

> All women, who come to deliver a child, should be met and taken by the gatekeeper immediately, without asking anything, both day and night. . . . If one does not want to show her face, it is allowed to her at all times. In the year of foundation, 5 children were born in the hospital opened 'for foundlings and homeless babies'. An infant born in that department was necessarily given to the Orphanage. (Lavrov 1983 cited by Loginov and Zainulina 2017)

Over time, obstetric institutions began to be perceived, however, as a relative norm for many city dwellers, including noble ladies (Mitsyuk, Belova, Pushkareva 2021). By the middle of the twentieth century, there had been a multiple increase in the number of maternity hospitals in Russia and childbirth became almost completely medicalised and went completely under the patronage of institutional medicine (Temkina 2014). The birth of a child in a medical institution was considered the accepted norm in society, at least in large cities (Mitsyuk and Pushkareva 2021). However, maternity facilities continued to be seen as a place of first care for the pregnant woman. The staffing levels show that obstetricians and gynaecologists dominated there and there was no 24-hour paediatric service.

The obstetric service went on actively developing during Soviet power. In 1929, the Motherhood and infancy protection homes were reformatted into so-called Women's consultations (antenatal clinics) (Novikov 2010), which shows the growing separation of paediatrics and obstetrics. After the Second World War and the adoption of a number of pronatalist directives, there was a steady increase in the birth rate and, as a result, the construction of new maternity hospitals. In 1987, in the region of our research, 74,087 births were recorded in the entire history of the region, which was the absolute maximum, while the number of obstetric beds was about 3,500 (Novikov 2010). At the same time, such medical areas as surgery and intensive care of newborns are developing in parallel, which results in a growing demand for paediatricians in those institutions. By that time, the process of division between adult and children's hospitals was finally completed. However, the presence of two completely different but inextricably linked patients in one institution – a mother and her newborn child – became a challenge for medical knowledge and organisations.

The place where it would be initially possible to combine adult and paediatric specialists (highly specialised) was, for example, the Pediatric Medical Institute, founded in 1925 as the Institute of Maternity and Infancy Protection. In 1968, the first resuscitation and intensive care unit for newborns (3 beds and 12 beds, respectively) for children with surgical pathology was opened there (Shabalov and Alexandrovichs 2018). However, the vast majority of obstetric institutions had no conditions for providing care to newborns in need of special treatment. The resources of university clinics also could not cover the needs of providing care to all pregnant women at risk. Besides, prenatal diagnostics of that time was not capable of diagnosing congenital malformations in utero; that is, medical professionals found out about the need for specialised care for newborns during or after childbirth.

There were several ways to solve this problem. The first was the expansion of existing university clinics, which already had both maternity wards and neonatal care ones. However, that could not cover all cases of complicated labour in the region. The second was the construction of a new type of institution, such as perinatal medical centres, where specialised medical care could be provided to both mother and child. Such a solution was assessed as the most efficient professional- and organisational-wise, but it required large resources and a change in the entire existing infrastructure, that is, the closure of many newly built maternity hospitals, relocation of surgeons, neurologists, cardiologists, ophthalmologists and other subspecialists from children's hospitals to new perinatal medical centres. And finally, the third way was to create an intermediary service that could combine the existing infrastructure of pregnancy and newborn care in the reanimation and advisory centre for newborns (NRAC). It was the latter option of the intermediate service that was implemented in the region and became decisive in the development of neonatal care in the region.

RESUSCITATION AND ADVISORY CENTRE (1980S)

One of the most important steps in the development of neonatal care in the region was the opening of a new children's hospital in 1977 (Order 888, 1977). It included 12 intensive care beds for newborns and 60 beds for the neonatal pathology department (16 of them for premature babies and 10 – for newborns with central nervous system disease). At that time, there were several small hospitals in the city. Mostly, they provided care and feeding for newborns and premature babies (Khazanov 1973). Since the founding of The Children's City Hospital, the centre for neonatal surgery and neonatology, both academically and practically, has moved from a university clinic to a large municipal hospital. The hospital began to develop malformation surgery and became a major training ground for medical personnel.

A Newborn Resuscitation and Advisory Centre (NRAC, later renamed as RAC, for consistency we use the modern acronym further) was opened at the hospital, where ambulance doctors worked, combining their practice in the neonatal intensive care unit with trips to maternity hospitals. Their task was to provide specialised care to children in maternity hospitals and, if necessary, transport them to general children's ones. The RAC system was formed in the early 1980s, and it has existed to this day, retaining the general principles of its work. It currently includes a consultant doctor, who performs round-the-clock monitoring and consultations of specialists from all the city's first and second-level medical institutions,[2] and three mobile teams, properly equipped for transporting newborns, including premature babies (the smallest surviving child transported by the RAC teams weighed 390g).

Over the past 40 years, neonatology has undergone revolutionary innovations that have significantly changed not only the outcomes and methods of treatment but also the perception of these patients among doctors. The field data showed that at the beginning of the existence of the RAC service, the attitude towards early premature babies (born before 28 weeks) was in many ways reminiscent of the period of the first shelter for premature babies in the early twentieth century. Until 1993, a live birth was defined as a child born at a gestational age of 28 weeks or more, weighing 1,000g or more, 35cm tall or more and who began to breathe after birth. Children with less body weight were included in the number of the living only if they lived 7 full days (168 hours). The birth of such a child was not considered as a birth and most often occurred in the gynaecological departments of adult hospitals, where newborns could not receive specialised care. If the child did not die in the first hours, then the existence of this child was reported to the RAC consultant, and a transport team (which, as a rule, did not include a doctor) left for him.

> Well, there were very few places [to take them to]. And you see, the thing is that they did not call those children 'children' from the very beginning. It was because when we started working, those children, they were not counted until the 10th day (in practice mostly until 7 days), and they were transferred from maternity hospitals. There were two medical cars [with doctors] and one the so-called 'microtransport' car [without a doctor]. It was even spelled out in the regulations that it had to be so. . . . And it was just them, nurses, who worked there, you see, we had just nurses, they were transporting all those children. (Doctor RAC 1, January 2023)

There were no doctors there because of several reasons. Firstly, as it was already mentioned, those children were considered to be 'late miscarriages', and they had to live 7 days in order to 'deserve' the status of a child. Secondly, at that time, the resuscitation teams did not have the necessary equipment at their disposal to provide specialised care, i.e. primarily respiratory support. Traveling around the gynaecological departments of various hospitals, the nurses 'collected' the surviving babies and took them to a small children's hospital, which was engaged in nursing premature babies. Judging by the descriptions of eyewitnesses, there were different attitudes towards early premature babies in different gynaecological departments – in some departments, the paramedics took the children wrapped and warmed, and in the others, they found them lying in 'boxes' or medical trays. Since those children did not actually have a legal status, the procedure for providing medical care to them was also not regulated, and much depended on the staff's personal attitude towards them.

> When we were just starting, there were childbirth in gynaecology, small children weighing up to nine hundred grammes, 900 grammes, up to a kilogram, who were called just 'foetus'. Until they lived for ten days (seven days), they had then to live for ten days in order to be referred to children. They weren't even

included in infant mortality. They needed to grow up to a kilogram so that later they could be officially transferred somewhere. Such children were registered with us for a very long time. As soon as there were more places in hospitals, we began to transfer them. That way. And those little ones, which were small, we then initially took them to the Nth hospital. There was no ventilation there. Nothing. We went to gynaecology units. You take him and he's cold, ugly. But some were okay at the first day, they were very good, so to speak, they had a large reserve. And it was already depleted quickly, melting, and they were not viable, as a rule. You know, besides, it was because, they were not counted and, so to speak, were not referred to as children, well, there was such an attitude. That's not for . . . (laughs wearily) Well, they were just put in the crib, and they lay there. If there was an incubator, of course, they put them in it. Well, the most important thing was respiratory support and 'Curosurf'. We didn't have it [at that time]. (Doctor RAC 1, January 2023)

Until the late 1980s, there was no intensive care unit in a hospital that specialised in nursing and treating early premature babies. Medical care was limited to appropriate care, nutrition and antimicrobial therapy. As nurses brought another premature baby to this hospital, they just wrote down his or her surname in a special hospital admissions register, and right there they saw that many of the previous ones had been 'crossed out':

Because it was, you know, once we were at [the location], that kind of thing. . . . There was a reception, [they were taking] those foetuses. He [a doctor] was sitting there like this and there was, well, a notebook. We wrote down what was in the record: the names and, of course, you can see there from the previous day that every second one there: 'Died, died'. That is, through one. Those, who were brought, the children, they were also there, I mean they have already been recorded. And so, he, so sad, says: 'Well, you brought me [them] here again. . . . As God wills, so it is'. (Nurse, RAC, January 2023)

Until a certain moment, the doctors of the resuscitation and advisory centre practically did not encounter patients from the 'foetus' category, providing neonatal care to children with congenital malformations, aspiration syndromes and infectious diseases that were more promising in terms of recovery and prognosis. It is worth noting that it was not an easy task given the absence of transport ventilators, endotracheal tubes and catheters:

That is, at first it was a complete nightmare. Well, I don't know, somehow, we brought someone. Pneumothoraxes were brought on manual ventilation. I remember N-maternity hospital. I was carrying him alone, here. Well, he arrived safely (she laughs). And they had diaphragmatic [Congenital diaphragmatic hernia], we brought different ones. Of course, some of the children remained in the hospital. And there was a completely different approach there.

> I mean they were saying: 'Take it away', and, of course, we took those children if possible. If we get him alive, it'll be great. So, he is lucky. But if we if we don't deliver him. . . . We didn't have any pressure gauges to measure the pressure. We determined the pressure even only by the pulse. (Doctor RAC 1, January 23)

> R: Well, at that time we had nothing to intubate a 500-gramme patient with. Earlier, when we started, we didn't have any endotracheal tubes, we made, excuse me, tubes from gas outlets. It was such a beautiful rubber tube. Well, they were cut off, like this one, the endotracheal tube should be bent at a certain angle. They were sterilised, and it happened that this tube stratified after multiple sterilisations, and already worked as a valve. (Doctor RAC 1, January 2023)

As will be shown a little further, technology has had a huge impact not only on the treatment of newborn patients but also on their perception within the medical community, being ahead of the law in this area.

By the end of the 1980s, a fairly stable system of inpatient care for newborns was taking shape. Four city hospitals were opened to provide care for children up to a month old: one specialised in surgical pathology, the second in premature babies and the other two were general hospitals. Those ones were supposed to provide assistance to newborns who were in obstetric institutions (there were more than a dozen in the city and the nearest suburbs). One of the main tasks of that time was to accurately assess the remote condition of a newborn. The maternity hospitals of that time had no intensive care units for newborns, ventilators, or qualified resuscitators. The RAC consultant doctor could have more than 20 children under his supervision, and he had to select the most needy and determine the level of neonatal care in order to send one of the two neonatal mobile teams there. To do this, it was necessary to come up with a language of communication between specialists with different levels of qualifications and experience. In this matter, they decided to rely on mathematicians and the cybernetic approach, which since the 1960s of the twentieth century had a special status in Russia (Rispoli, 2015). For example, numerous ACS (automated control systems) were created everywhere, including in the medical field. The essence of this approach to the registration of newborns was as follows: the risk of a fatal outcome was calculated on the basis of the assessment of one of the signs (medical indicator). In fact, it was a scale of threat measurement, which a questionnaire was made from later. It was called the 'formalised information form' (FIF). One of the FIF developers, a resuscitator, spoke in her interview about the implementation of this approach as follows:

> we had a computer programme called AWP or an automated workplace. It was never completed to the end, but there was an idea of (making a decision)

> according to these coefficients. . . . They (superiors) came to us at the conference and asked, why this or that child was not translated with such a coefficient, why. But later all this subsided and we found out about those coefficients. This was good as a tool – it helped to understand! But at the end, it was the doctor, who was responsible anyway. . . . The ideas were good, everyone was taught at the maternity hospital. We all worked kinda in the same way, understood all those meanings. (Interview with a Doctor, RAC 2, February 2023)

This questionnaire and the formalisation of severity condition assessment led to very important changes; that is, many institutions with specialists of different skill levels were able to speak the same language, describing the signs of the disease or the severity of the condition. While transmitting information about the child's condition, the maternity hospital doctor not only reported the main indicators that doctors were guided by when assessing the state of health (pulse, respiratory rate and pressure), but also systematically described the colour of the skin, breathing patterns, the degree of activity, the level of consciousness of the newborn, that is, he systematically pronounced and assessed the current state of the child. What was originally dry statistics and mathematics turned into a manual for a thorough examination of the child with a detailed description of his or her appearance and subsequent transmission of that information at a distance. Despite the fact that the original idea of automation through scoring actually failed, this form lasted about 15 years as a successful communication tool between doctors of different medical organisations:

> And they didn't finish it [software] to the end, but there was an idea about what those coefficients [could help to do], but the authors believed that they had come up with those coefficients. They came to us at the conference and asked why a child was not transferred with such a coefficient, why. But later it all subsided, and those coefficients were good as a tool because they helped to understand; and on the other hand, you can't legally hold those (FIFs[3]) responsible. I mean the doctor is responsible anyway. They wanted to monitor the entire list of patients on the screen according to those coefficients so that you could immediately see how serious they were, not all, but serious. Some kind of coefficient rolled over, you could click it and immediately you had that data.
>
> And further continues: I mean we spoke the same language, the same language. When new doctors came to the maternity hospital, it was terrible. They called and did not understand what was happening with the child, what, how, whether he was serious or something else. It was a total mess. But when they started working according to those signs, everything became much easier. (Interview with a doctor, RAC 2, February 2023)

In addition to the formal tasks of treating and transporting newborns, another very important implicit function of the advisory centre was revealed over the time, that is, informal external control. Medical structures (departments, hospitals) are often closed institutions not only in relation to patients but also in relation to any outsider agents, including external medical organisations or medical schools, being on the one hand a narrow professional sphere of activity and on the other hand a rather vulnerable area with high legal risks. Medical organisations have historically been studied and considered to be closed systems, which the monopoly of knowledge and expertise was unevenly distributed in (Goffman 1961; Freidson 1988). In many ways, Soviet health care institutions could also be considered quasi-total institutions, which had limited access of relatives to the patients, and the patients themselves had no opportunity to influence the course of diagnosis and treatment. Even communication with medical personnel was restricted (Temkina et al. 2021, 102). Those properties of medicine are still manifested in some respects even at the present time, in the area of emergency and resuscitation care in particular, where access to patients' relatives is still largely limited. Public campaigns and statements by the expert community about the need to overcome this closeness partly led to results. For example, in 2020, a law on 'open resuscitation' was adopted (Order of the Ministry of Health, 2020). However, resuscitation often remains without external control from the patients' relatives and the public eye.

Another global problem of medicine is medical errors. They occur in all countries, regardless of the level of the health system, and are one of the leading causes of death (Rodziewicz and Hipskind 2020). In Russia, it is hard to evaluate or assess this problem accurately since there are no exact statistics on this issue. In 2019, the Investigative Committee of Russia received about 6.5 thousand complaints about improper provision of medical care (Sergeeva and Zinenko 2021). But those figures rather reflect the level of legal awareness of citizens, their alertness, or distrust in the healthcare system [than true figures]. In addition, due to the closeness of medical units, not all errors become known. At best, the identified errors and shortcomings become the subject of analysis within the departments (collegially), less often – at commissions of various levels. Although medical errors were not the subject of the study, this topic repeatedly came up in the course of field research as the doctors of the RAC constantly discussed the patients they treated in different hospitals, recalculated the dosages of drugs in case of their incorrect calculation, corrected the treatment in case of incorrect diagnosis of critical conditions. The presence of an 'outside' doctor, even if he or she is well-known, is often perceived as a kind of inspection. Anthropologists, who observed the interaction between a RAC doctor and a maternity ward neonatologist, described their first impression the following way:

she said in such a high voice, as if justifying and at the same time with feigned-confident intonation that he had normal pressure. In general, her intonation seemed interesting to me. She often happened to speak so confidently, raising her voice, giving comments about the treatment and the condition of the child, answering A's questions. By doing so, she kind of constructed her confidence and competence, her status. And sometimes it sounded as if she justified herself at the same time. (Diary of observations, November 2020)

When transferring newborns, RAC doctors review medical documentation, conduct their own examination and assessment of the condition. Often, as a result of discussion, therapy is adjusted and the severity is reassessed. Unlike emergency services, which transfer older children or adults from time to time, RAC doctors work daily in the same medical institutions, become well-connected, gain trust or distrust, they know personally each doctor with whom they interact. In an interview, to the question: 'Do you know all the heads?', the RAC consultant physician answers:

[I knew] the heads, of course, and the doctors of the maternity hospital. [I recognised them] – by their voices. [I knew] what expect from them, who told a lie, who worked well, who was something else. [. . .] Even that influenced whether [we had to] send a team or not. Or [we'd better] agree on treatment, do this, that, something different. [. . .] Well, as a new person appeared there, in the maternity hospital, a head called us and asked, if there was anything, to immediately respond to any stupidity and go to the [doctor's] call. If the doctor asked to leave, it meant to go for a consultation. (Interview with a Doctor RAC 2, February 2023)

As the neonatal service was developing, the doctors of the mobile teams did a lot of work to train the staff, they went out for the most insignificant reasons, turning the hospitals included in the RAC system into inpatient departments open for observation and hospitalisation: Technological Breakthrough (1990s)

They [newborns] could be staying there from several days up to a week. And we needed, well, firstly, to examine some according to the plan, to sanitise the others, [because] they couldn't do that there, in maternity hospitals, and [we decided] who needed to be urgently transferred. (Interview with a Doctor, RAC 2, February 2023)

This practice continues to this day, despite a significantly increased level of care. There is an intensive care unit in every city maternity hospital, and qualified neonatal resuscitators work there. The staff of the RAC provided neonatal care in other institutions, which helped to 'study' the inner specifics of the work in each department, that is, their strengths and weaknesses, organisational features, material capabilities and resources. The RAC was not empowered to impose sanctions, so the service did not pose 'a threat' to institutions, which allowed doctors to observe the real situation inside the departments.

TECHNOLOGICAL BREAKTHROUGH (1990S)

The advent and implementation of neonatal ventilators in maternity hospitals and on ambulances that transported children from maternity hospitals to paediatric hospitals has resulted in significant progress in the care of newborns. The real breakthrough, however, was the use of surfactant.[4] If in the early 1980s survival among children weighing less than 1,500g was 65–70%, by the end of the 1990s, it increased to 85% (Lyubimenko, Pankratov and Mostovoy, 2005). At the same time, there was a steady increase in children born weighing less than 1,000g. If in 1991 they were 144.1 per 10,000 live births, five years later this figure increased by 26% (Lyubimenko, Pankratov and Mostovoy, 2005). Surfactants began to be used in clinical practice in the region in 1993, and since that time the attitude towards premature babies weighing less than 1,000g has begun to change:

> At that time, premature babies were a big problem for us. Of course, it was very disappointing, when you couldn't help a child of 2.5 kilogrammes. That kind of thing. [It happened] because until the 1990s we had, in general, neither manual ventilation devices, nor adequate infusion therapy, there was none of that. The most important thing was missing, that curosurf.[5] [We didn't have] surfactant, [we couldn't] make up for the deficiency of surfactant to make up for the deficiency in those children. Like this. Of course, with the advent of artificial ventilation devices and curosurf, well, sure, it has already become noticeable how much this progress has been made. Yeah. And, of course, we have learned to work with those children both in terms of infusion therapy and some kind of respiratory support. (Interview with a Doctor RAC 1, January 2023)

> Well, at that time, there was no surfactant there, I mean curosurf. So in general, children [remained connected] for a long time, if they could not be on respiratory support, on a large percentage of oxygen. That kind of thing. . . . With the appearance [of curosurf] it became noticeable: as you enter this curosurf, they quickly leave the device and are transferred, and everything is fine. (Doctor RAC 1, January 2023)

A major contribution to the development of neonatology in the region was the Heart to Heart Foundation programme, which helped to exchange experience with American colleagues in the field of heart disease surgery and nursing children with extremely low body weight. The history of this fund began with the fall of the Iron Curtain, when one of the Soviet translators, working at the festival of Soviet American cinema, turned to one of the American clinics for help. Her daughter was operated on at the Oakland Heart Clinic by Dr Nilos Young. In those days, open heart surgery was not performed on children in the Soviet Union. The case received publicity and was followed by letters from the Soviet Union, asking for help. The charitable medical foundation Heart to Heart was formed that way. In 1989, about 20 specialists arrived in Russia. They were doctors, nurses and medical technicians, led by paediatric cardiologist Stanley Higashino and cardiac surgeon Nilas Young. They brought instruments, equipment and medicines and for several months operated on children together with Russian colleagues, teaching them. Subsequently, several times a year, volunteer doctors from U.S. hospitals came back and trained medical staff in the treatment and diagnosis of heart defects and nursing premature babies (Heart to Heart, 2023). This experience, with the early introduction of new technologies, allowed the region to become one of the leaders in Russia in terms of low levels of infant mortality for many years and changed the perception of doctors regarding the prospects for very premature babies.

STATIONARY CARE AND COMPETITION (1990S–2010S)

By the late 1980s and the early 1990s, a system of four paediatric hospitals was formed in the region. It provided care for newborn children, and each hospital occupied its own niche. As was already said, the history of hospital care for newborns began in 1901, when the first shelter for premature babies was opened. This shelter moved many times to different addresses and eventually became part of one of those four hospitals, continuing to provide care for premature babies. Each of the four hospitals had its own peculiarity. One specialised in very premature babies, the second in surgical pathology, the third focused on mother-child interaction and the possibility of joint stay of newborn patients and their mothers and the fourth managed to create almost ideal epidemiological conditions. The doctors who led the departments of newborns were representatives of the same medical school and constituted one professional community. Therefore, the experience, gained in the work of existing institutions, was largely taken into account when new hospitals and departments were planned to open:

> Well, firstly, we had one leader, who supervised us – N [the former chief freelance neonatologist of the region]. All these ideas were his . . . if pediatricians (neonatologists) were supervised by Shabalov, we (neonatal resuscitators) were supervised by Lyubimenko [the former chief freelance neonatologist of the region].

> Therefore, we had no discrepancies with either the Pediatric hospital A or the Pediatric hospital B. (Head of one of the first NICU[6] in Russia, February 2023)

New institutions also became places for organisational innovations. For example, it was the implementation of the principle of co-habitation of mother and child, which was a significant challenge for healthcare organisers of that period, since there were no precedents there:

> We suffered so much with the mothers at the previous hospital. . . . Together with Lyubimenko [the former chief freelance neonatologist of the region], we planned it all somehow, built it, so that we allocated a lot of mother beds. Maternal beds are not children's, they need to be fed somehow, some kind of hygiene should be, I mean showers, toilets, a lot of things to do, food, [because] they are adults. It's like a maternity hospital here . . . forty newborns and somewhere around thirty-five mothers. . . . The problem is huge with those children (mothers), and all the publications say: mother-child, mother-child. You can't do anything without a mother. Firstly, this is a good control for nurses, it is very important that mom is always nearby. She cannot mess around there, do some unknown thing, or come late, or something like that [and forget about] a child. [When mom is nearby] she must come. (Head of one of the first NICU in Russia, February 2023)

The specialisation of hospitals at that time had different reasons. On the one hand, organisational traditions (institutional continuity) played an important role; for example, one of the hospitals, being the successor to the previously mentioned shelter for premature babies, had accumulated experience in nursing premature babies over the years and subsequently retained this specialisation. Its doctors made a great contribution to the nursing of very premature babies. They developed this area of care for newborns even before the widespread use of mechanical ventilation. Before the opening of perinatal medical centres, children weighing up to a kilogram were born, as a rule, in gynaecological departments and did not receive any resuscitation or specialised care after birth. If such newborns did not die during the first hours, they were taken to the hospital. When the question arose of organising a resuscitation and intensive care unit for premature babies, the service was transferred to the newly renovated building where doctors continued to nurse those children, but it was already within the framework of the intensive care unit.

As for the surgical hospital, it had other reasons for the subspeciality. In conditions of a relative shortage of beds, the surgical hospital could not afford to occupy a bed for a long time with an extremely low birth weight child (which, as a rule, required long-term observation and treatment):

D. (former chief freelance neonatologist) did not allow extreme newborns to be taken (children weighing less than 1,000 grammes at birth), as he was afraid that there would be no room for surgery. (Interview with a Head of NICU at a surgical hospital, March 2023)

At the initial stage, the competition between those hospitals looked like a professional competition in terms of success indicators:

What is competition for newborns? It means who will take whom. In principle, we always knew that we were taking such a piece (from another fragment: we did not take less than 1,2 kilos, 1,3 kilos). The other took the smallest ones and all the surgery. Competition was not for patients, but for the result. The result was important for us. (Head of one of the first NICU in Russia, February 2023)

Well, he was envious, he came from the large hospital (about one of the heads of neonatal resuscitation). He also believed that he could (organise the department) and he focused precisely on sterility. (Head of one of the first NICU in Russia, February 2023)

Subsequently, as market mechanisms of regulation penetrated the healthcare sector, competition became more intense, as it required hospitals to adapt to changing conditions and develop to maintain the flow of patients. Over time, each of the paediatric hospitals, dealing with (children having) certain pathologies, has formed its own treatment approaches. Some hospitals were distinguished by more aggressive treatment, some less so. This led to the fact that the doctors of the RAC, in addition to the specialisation of the hospital, began to take into account conditions of patients and did not take severe ones to hospitals, where more sparing therapeutic approaches were used, which often led to death. Besides, the surgical hospital began to take children with extremely low body weight:

At some point we looked at the statistics and saw that in the XX [hospital specialising in premature babies] children died. This group is characterised by surgical problems – 'bellies' and 'ducts',[7] so we began to take more of them [extremely low birth weight newborns]. (Head of NICU at the surgical hospital, March 2023)

A combination of a new coronavirus infection, a sharp decline in the birth rate in the region, and the inability of the hospital administration to respond in a timely manner to changing conditions resulted in the closing of two neonatal departments in four hospitals by the beginning of 2022. The need for intensive care beds was covered by the expansion of the intensive care unit of the surgical hospital, which made it possible to route all children with extremely low body weight (ELBW) to the hospital that could provide surgical care:

> they had a lot of good ideas, for example, a small operating room, round-the-clock x-rays, they planned completely different boxes. But the head doctor did nothing to change the situation so that they could continue to treat children with extremely low body weight, and everything withered . . . although they had good results, the children felt fine, with good eyes without BPD [bronchopulmonary dysplasia]. (Interview with a head of NICU at the surgical hospital, March 2023)

LEGAL BACKGROUND ON NEONATOLOGY

According to the WHO definition, a live birth is

> the complete expulsion or extraction from its mother of a product of conception, irrespective of the duration of pregnancy, which, after such separation, breathes or shows any other evidence of life, such as beating of the heart, pulsation of the umbilical cord, or definite movement of voluntary muscles, whether or not the umbilical cord has been cut or the placenta is attached. (World Health Organisation 2010, 151)

Most countries of the world use this definition with some clarifications and additions that determine the legal status of a newborn in a specific legal and social context. Despite the huge progress in the field of nursing and treatment of premature newborns, the application of the proposed criteria to children born at terms up to 22 weeks does not allow to count on a favourable outcome regarding their future health and quality of life, although modern methods of treatment can help to maintain the functions of their life support systems for a long time. Therefore, the proposed definition is rather an ethical guideline or a reserve for the future (Volodin 2008). Nevertheless, in 1992 and 2012, adjustments were made to the laws, bringing the live birth criteria in Russia closer to those proposed by WHO. Preparations were complex and included the construction of perinatal centres (Government Decree 2007, 2013), the implementation of pronatalist measures to support young families (Rivkin-Fish 2010; Chernova 2013), as well as changes in professional standards and procedures for providing medical care to pregnant women, women in childbirth and newborns (Decree of the Ministry 2011, 2012a, b, 2020).

The measures and laws not only changed the legal status of newborns, the organisation of neonatal care and professional approaches to the diagnosis, treatment and resuscitation of newborn patients but also created a number of new ethical challenges. Resuscitation of children at 22 weeks of gestation is not strictly mandatory in most countries of the world; however, Russia is one of the few exceptions, since resuscitation is mandatory there according to the new live birth criteria (Korobeev and Shirshov 2020). Accordingly, each formal change in the live birth criteria significantly changed the organisation of neonatal care and professional practices of newborn care.

In 1992, two orders (Order of the Ministry of Health 1992; Resolution of the State Statistics Committee 1992) introduced new criteria into the practice of recording live and still births. Those changes concerned medical statistics, that is, only children weighing more than 1,000g were registered in the authorised bodies for registering children (registry offices), or from 500 to 999g if they lived for more than 168 hours (i.e., 1 week). This made it possible to change the previously accepted routing, after which women with gestations up to 28 weeks began to go to maternity hospitals instead of gynaecological departments, where newborns had the opportunity to receive medical care. At the same time, if such a child died within 168 hours, he or she was considered stillborn and did not fall into part of the statistical data. Such legal duality left a certain level of freedom for local doctors regarding the treatment and resuscitation of such patients. Statistical data from different regions of Russia from that period confirm this conclusion. The professional community still called those children 'foetuses', but technological possibilities and the advent of surfactant significantly increased their chances of recovery.

In 2012, according to the Order of the Ministry of Health and Social Development (Order of the Ministry of Health and Social Development 2011), the birth criteria were again changed. A live birth began to be considered the appearance of a child at a gestational age of 22 weeks or more, weighing 500g or more, and 25cm tall or more. Such formal transformations led primarily to changes in demographic indicators, such as an increase in the birth rate and perinatal losses, as well as to organisational changes in the neonatal service, that is, an increase in the number of beds for newborns and paediatric beds, a reorganisation of the obstetric service, the workload of which increased with the expansion of the contingent and the number of obstetric patients (who were considered gynaecological until 2012) (Starodubov and Sukhanova 2013).

It is worth noting that in the region under study, new live birth criteria practically did not change the statistical indicators of the work of the neonatological service because, firstly, since 2010, the region of research was one of two regions that had implemented a pilot programme to modernise neonatology, and, secondly, by the time of those legislative changes, a certain system of care for newborns had already been established in the city, which made it possible to successfully nurse premature babies, including children with extremely low body weight. Next follows a description of what exactly those and other key features of neonatal care currently consist of.

THE CURRENT STRUCTURE OF NEONATAL CARE IN THE REGION OF RESEARCH

It is necessary to mention that neonatal care is still very strongly integrated into the maternity obstetric service as a whole. Therefore, some of the features of the organisation, financing and regulation of neonatology are predetermined by the way obstetric and gynaecological care in Russia is arranged. In particular, researchers note the very pronounced medicalisation and technologisation of this care (Temkina et al. 2022; Temkina 2014), as well as the fact that this entire system attracts close attention from various government agencies due to the pronatalist nature of social and demographic policies (Rivkin-Fish 2010; Chernova 2013) and the statist turn in the nature of the management of the social sphere in general, which occurred after 2006 (Cook 2011; Tarasenko 2018; Matveev and Novkunskaya 2021).

Neonatal care and medical care for women during pregnancy and childbirth share the routing system built over the past ten years, which makes it possible to assess the risks of complications and pathologies during monitoring pregnancy. It helps to hospitalise women with a certain level of risk of complications in institutions that are adequately equipped to provide necessary medical care. The system of routing pregnant women was built and exists mostly thanks to large technologically equipped perinatal centres, as well as a rather significant centralisation of obstetric care within each region.

At the moment, the three-level system of care for pregnant women, women in labour and newborns is regulated by order of the Ministry of Health No. 1130n (Order of the Ministry 2020). It assumes that in the regions there are small institutions of the first level (no more than 500 births per year), located in maximum accessibility for residents of rural areas and areas remote from the centres. Such maternity wards are prepared for only physiological childbirth; they do not provide a round-the-clock stay of a doctor, that is, an obstetrician-gynaecologist, a neonatologist and an anaesthesiologist-resuscitator, and all complex cases must be sent to institutions of the second and third levels. Obstetric hospitals of the second level are properly equipped to provide more complex medical care and should have resuscitation and intensive care units (NICU) in their structure for both women and newborns.

Third-level institutions are the most technically equipped obstetric hospitals, which are also divided into two categories: A-category maternity hospitals and perinatal centres must have a department for the pathology of newborns and premature babies (stage II of nursing), as well as an obstetric remote consultative centre with a telemedicine department, including mobile obstetric teams. Perinatal centres of the third level B (which already have federal rather than regional subordination) provide specialised medical care (including high-tech) for women during pregnancy, childbirth, the postpartum period and newborns. Such institutions not only provide medical care but also develop new methods for diagnosing and treating obstetric and neonatal pathologies, as well as monitor and provide organisational and methodological support to all other obstetric hospitals (Ibid).

However, even the federal perinatal centres do not always provide newborns with the full range of specialised care. Therefore, hospitalisation of newborns requiring specialised care in multidisciplinary paediatric hospitals should be organised within each region. The routing of this profile of medical care is regulated under the Order of the Ministry of Health No. 921n. However, in fact, it is organised within each region differently, as it depends on the configuration of the available obstetric and paediatric hospitals, as well as how the service responsible for transferring children from obstetric institutions to others is arranged and structured.

It is also worth noting that, according to the law, obstetric care for pregnant women is free of charge, covered by mandatory health insurance (MHI). The route of a pregnant woman today is in many ways reminiscent of the route in Soviet times, that is, during pregnancy, women must be observed in antenatal clinics by an obstetrician-gynaecologist, and they must undergo mandatory screenings once a trimester to diagnose possible intrauterine pathology. Then women enter the maternity hospital either with the onset of labour or, as planned, if a certain method of delivery is required. The commercial sector of obstetrics is developing rapidly, but mostly women either use free services or combine MHI services with commercial ones (paying for a separate room, the possibility of a partner being present, getting to know the obstetrician-gynaecologist and midwife in advance). A small number of private maternity hospitals (mostly located in metropolitan areas) also have a neonatal service, but they are designed more for uncomplicated cases. In particular, there are four private maternity hospitals in the study region. They are also included in the RAC system, and in case of complications or an uneven course of the disease, newborns from private maternity hospitals can be routed to one of the two paediatric hospitals in the city. Another reason for the transfer may be a material factor because the stay of a newborn in the intensive care unit is not always covered by the delivery contract.

If the baby is born healthy and does not require specialised care, after discharge from the maternity hospital, he or she is observed by the district paediatrician and/or patronage nurse. All subsequent examinations, vaccinations and screenings take place in children's clinics. There are other institutional trajectories for children with clinically or socially complicated circumstances. Those patients who require high-tech care due to some disease are hospitalised in specialised paediatric hospitals. Patients with organ pathology or requiring differential diagnosis, but without direct threat to life, can spend quite a long time in neonatal pathology departments. From there, if necessary, patients with an unfavourable clinical prognosis are transferred to palliative services, or if parents refuse the child, the newborn is sent to the children's home.

Thus, numerous specialists in different types of organisations are responsible for the health of the child at different stages of his or her development. In practice, this situation may lead to a lack of continuity of care, families often face inconsistencies in the approaches of antenatal clinics, private clinics, specialised centres, state maternity hospitals, paediatric hospitals and children's clinics. Different medical professionals, even within the same speciality, have different backgrounds and resources, and local protocols vary across hospitals and departments within them. Working in each of these different organisational contexts requires complex coordination and is often manually managed (Temkina et al. 2022); that is, it requires a lot of negotiation between different specialists and employees of different organisations. As a result, different institutions are often poorly coordinated with each other and sometimes have conflicting views on the same issues or aspects of pregnancy, childbirth and newborn care.

So, neonatal care in the region is built into this general legal and organisational framework, however, due to historical and other local features, it also has a number of differences from other regions. In general, the system of care for newborns in this region consists of a lot of obstetric hospitals and includes two federal centres that provide neonatal care mainly to patients from other regions of Russia and are not included in the city routing (3,886 births per year [hereinafter, the date given are at the time of conducting the study]), and 19 institutions conditionally included in the RAC system (47,754 births per year), which consist of two institutes, seven city maternity hospitals, four obstetric departments in multidisciplinary hospitals, a city perinatal centre and four private clinics. Newborns can be transferred from these 19 institutions to one of the two city children's hospitals (97 intensive care beds and 244 neonatal pathology beds), one of which houses another separate care sector – a neonatal resuscitation and advisory centre responsible for transporting and routing newborns between all medical institutions in the region.

About 50,000 children are born in the region every year, and about 10% of births occur to residents from other regions, another 10% – to residents of the adjacent region and another 10% – to foreign citizens. About 4,000 patients a year are transported by the RAC service from obstetric institutions, of which 1,500 are children in need of maintaining vital functions (lung ventilation). All newborns can be conditionally divided into two categories – children in need of resuscitation care (or intensive observation) and children with a pathology that is not life-threatening but requires treatment and observation in a hospital. Depending on their condition, they receive care either in the intensive care unit or in the neonatal pathology unit. A few years ago, such medical care was provided in four paediatric hospitals, but now, only two remain due to an annual decrease in the number of births and a surplus of neonatal beds. Two other hospitals have been converted to paediatric and palliative care centres (according to a visiting chief neonatologist's expert interview). Approximately 10% of newborns require medical supervision and approximately 5.5–5.7% are born prematurely, very preterm or underweight, which is about 2,800–2,900 newborns per year. There are also several catamnesis rooms and rehabilitation departments where children can get assistance after the main treatment. Rehabilitation includes not only medical help, but also assistance in acquiring household and social skills. However, there is no single general programme for helping children who have had perinatal complications, and each department creates its own treatment standards.

In this chapter, we have described in detail the field of our study, taking into account the historical past and the current arrangement of the neonatal care system. The system of neonatal care in the region clearly shows the isolation of three sectors of inpatient neonatal care. The further content of the book will be related to the position of the newborn child in these three sectors.

NOTES

1. A baby is considered to be mature if born from 37 to 41 weeks of gestation.
2. The hospitals of the first level are hospitals that do not involve the treatment of newborns, the second-level hospitals are maternity hospitals that involve neonatal treatment and obstetric departments of multidisciplinary hospitals (22 departments for 2023 – data from the report of the chief freelance neonatologist).
3. Formalised information form (blank).
4. A medicine that keeps the lungs working well to prevent breathing problems.
5. The trade name of the most common surfactant used in Russia.
6. Neonatal intensive care unit.
7. Open ductus arteriosus is a congenital heart defect that results in the abnormal flow of blood from the aorta to the pulmonary artery. Ballies is slang for necrotising enterocolitis.

Chapter 2

In Searching for the Point of View

REFLECTIONS ON THE MULTIPLE ROLES OF THE RESEARCHERS

Co-author Artemiy: Physician

In a natural science environment, the researcher's position rarely requires explanation – the object of knowledge in biomedicine is material and objectified: it can be seen, counted, measured and so on. In the case of evidence-based medicine, the researcher's position requires depersonalisation and sort of 'self-blinding' (double-blind placebo-controlled trial) rather than explanation. However, like any concept, evidence-based medicine has its limitations and contextual variations (Borozdina 2023). Sometimes, the more carefully we design a study, the more distant it becomes from the reality in which the practitioner works. In order for the results obtained in laboratory settings to be applied in real-life practice, we need to bring real-life conditions closer to the laboratory (Latour and Woolgar 2013), which is not always possible in the context of medical practice.

Before I encountered the social sciences and their research methods, I worked as a physician for 13 years, and the positivist approach seemed to be the only possible means of cognition in medicine. Therefore, my encounter with sociology caused a sense of confusion, primarily because of the number of perspectives and variables with which the social sciences approach the object under study. In addition, the results of sociological research do not always have obvious practical value, they are descriptive in nature, which on the one hand complements the picture of reality, but on the other hand, at the same time, complicates it. Despite the abovementioned 'shortcomings', it is medical sociology and anthropology that come closest to answering the question of why 'pure laboratory' knowledge is not always easy to apply in practice. After all, treatment is not only about the use of medical knowledge; it is also about the interactions of people in different legal, bureaucratic and political circumstances.

Despite my experience in sociological and ethnographic research, I was still a practising physician and therefore always remained part of the research field, which had a certain impact on my perspective in field research. Self-observation became an important tool for me (on self-observation as a method see: Rodriguez and Ryave 2002), but in the process of collecting and analysing the material, I could not always detach myself enough, continuing to search for practical value in all observations and thinking about how to do my work better, thus acting in the mode of a 'doctor'. In doing so, I realised that the value of knowledge cannot always be defined only in terms of its utilitarian worth. The background of a physician sometimes narrowed the perspective, resulting in the dropping out of important details – everyday minutiae that were perceived as something ordinary and familiar, but still could harbour answers to research questions and highlight such topics as patient perspective, emotional labour and signs of colleague burnout. On the other hand, a medical background allows one to get into places where a 'person from the outside' can hardly penetrate, and if they do, they will not understand what they have seen – glances, casual utterances, omissions, rudeness and so on, all of which cannot be correctly interpreted without knowing the long history preceding the observed situation.

One of the peculiarities of our field was its heterogeneity – the observations have taken place on the territory of many medical organisations, each of which has its own local peculiarities, understanding of which also requires a long immersion in this environment. In this situation, my position of a complete 'insider' fitted best not only for entering the field but also for consulting fellow researchers. As a university student studying sociological and anthropological texts related to medicine, I sometimes felt like a 'native' being told how his tribe really lived. The main problem with this perception was that I always wanted to explain to the researcher the logic of medical behaviour, but the 'researcher' left it out of the question. For me, it was a matter of principle because, from my point of view, leaving medical aspects out of the equation multiplied the researchers' (or readers') interpretation of the data unnecessarily or vice versa reduced it to a statement of fact that hung in the air with the question 'what next?' This is by no means a criticism of social science, but it merely shows the limitations of a particular scientific approach. In classic works of ethnography, the issue of taking a 'fresh' look and at the same time immersing oneself in an environment was addressed through the means of extensive, prolonged field research – scholars lived and studied tribes and communities for years, gradually moving from the status of 'stranger' to a 'friend' or 'insider' (see the methodological discussion on the complexities of these positions and how it can change over time; see Powdermaker 1966; Humphrey 2007; Kersetter 2012; Dwyer and Buckle 2009; Breen 2007). Contemporary scholars in modern research projects do not always have such a huge time resource to enter the research field, compared, say, to Margaret Mead. A multidisciplinary approach is one way to address this limitation.

When I conducted my first joint observations with sociologists and anthropologists, it was immediately apparent how the underlying experience was reflected in the content of the diary entries. This effect was reinforced by the varying degrees of involvement of the observers. In the course of my professional duties and parallel field noting, I focused on key issues from a therapeutic point of view, leaving out peripheral medical and other routine details. An external observer, not knowing the intricacies of internal processes, followed what was happening from the outside, paying attention to social interactions rather than professional ones. This significantly enriched the field material. The next advantage of multidisciplinarity was the issue of interpretation of the observations obtained, namely the possibility of triangulation in the interpretation of the data obtained, on the part of a sociologist, an anthropologist and a medical professional. Each of us has a different perspective, and the challenge becomes to find the point at which these perspectives intersect. In the process of collecting material, I noticed how my position in the field influenced the focus of the research, which required some adjustment. Thus, the first diary entries were more like a medical staff's recording of the therapeutic process. The inclusion of an anthropologist and a sociologist as external observers allowed the focus to shift to the social interaction of the medical staff with each other and with patients. This was also applicable to the collaborative interviews, where I often engaged in a professional dialogue with the interviewer, rather than allowing the interviewee to develop their thoughts at a full scale. On the other hand, it was easy for me to navigate through the terminology, people and events that were mentioned in the interviews, which made it easier for everyone to work with the material. Being a part of the field under study, I repeatedly noticed how my fellow researchers looked at the 'showcases' intended for women-patients, which can be described by the well-known proverb 'not all that glitters is gold':

> We pass by maternity wards, each with its own original and unusual name. We enter the intensive care unit – it is quite spacious, bright, the windows overlook the courtyard, there's a lot of new equipment. There is only one patient, and the staff immediately introduces him as 'this is our Vasya'. (Diary of participant observations, maternity hospital, June 2023)

This is how the researcher saw the intensive care unit in one of the city's private maternity hospitals. In the same diary, we can see a description of the municipal maternity hospital, which was also the field research site that day:

> On the same floor, just through the door we enter the pediatric intensive care unit – it is newer and looks neater, although it is obvious that it is not very richly equipped and furnished (part of the ceiling tiles are coming off, the furniture and equipment look worn-out). The whole RAC team with the incubator goes into the ward – local staff comes in with them, there is no room left, as the intensive care ward is quite small, so I stay in the corridor). (Diary of participant observations, maternity hospital, June 2023)

Even from this brief description, when comparing a private and a municipal institution, the advantages of the latter seem obvious to an outside observer. In the case of the former, there are spacious wards, a lot of equipment; in the case of the latter, there is no place to turn around, and the equipment and furniture are old. But the paradox of the situation is that the described city hospital was much better equipped, and its therapeutic and diagnostic capabilities were wider. This once again convinced me of the importance of securing an 'insider' in any social research. Where there are no other research tools besides the personal gaze and speculations, it is extremely important to guard against erroneous conclusions.

In this respect, the multidisciplinary composition of the research team allowed us to correct each other in the process of collecting and analysing the material.

Co-author Anna: Anthropologist

I joined the study as an observer in early 2020 when it became clear that our co-author was having some difficulty in negotiating the boundaries between the immersion of a physician and the detachment of a social researcher. Beyond my natural anthropological curiosity, I was driven by the idea that my external gaze at the context under study, unclouded by medical optics, would help to actualise those details that had escaped our co-author's attention. The task seemed to be successful: my focus during fieldwork was on the communication between medical staff that the co-author could not notice, firstly due to his immersion in the process of treatment and filling out medical documents, and secondly because it represented a familiar routine difficult for him to single out and record in his diary. Thus, in my diaries, I have largely emphasised communication with the child and the emotional assessments addressed to her or him. Partly, this focus is related to my previous research experience: in my first anthropological project, I studied the frames of communication with severely disabled children in an orphanage and the symbolic classifications of children that existed in the perceptions of the staff who worked with them (Klepikova and Utekhin 2010). In the present research, I was interested in the degree of subjectivity given to a resuscitated baby, what it depends on, and how it relates to their medical status.

For an anthropologist, since the first classical studies (Malinowski 1922), participant observation has been the leading research method. Of course, there are anthropological projects based only on interviews or document analysis, but it is participant observation that is the gold standard of anthropology. At the same time, anthropological methodology implies reflection on the levels and facets of inclusion in the community under study and the degree of the anthropologist's participation in its life. Thus, if there is no question about the level of inclusion of our co-author-physician, I could hardly be called a full-fledged participant in the process of transporting a newborn baby. To some extent, I was more of a non-participant observer, as I was not part of the group under study (I am not a medical professional) and was not involved in any way in the work of the team; that is, I did not share their activities with my informants. My role in the field was, firstly, to communicate spontaneously with the transport team members and, secondly, to observe the work of the team and surrounding events during the child stabilisation process.

As an anthropologist usually working as a participant observer, I am used to being included in activities that are part of my informants' lives – for example, in the project I referred to above, I worked as a volunteer in an orphanage. In the context of high-tech medicine, such inclusion is unimaginable for a non-medical person, and I felt uncomfortable in the role of a 'disengaged' observer, being unaccustomed to it. Nevertheless, on subsequent field trips in 2023, my degree of involvement with the brigade began to increase. I intuitively tried to help roll the cart with the incubator on it or hold the doors for it to pass through, I dared to talk to moms the way the medical staff did (e.g., asking what the mom named the baby), and once I was even trusted to push a couple of buttons on the monitor and hold the infusion machine. My hands were shaking for fear of doing something wrong, but such a gesture meant symbolic inclusion as 'one of the kin'. In addition, in my diaries, I described what concerned the team in terms of inclusive pronouns: 'our' baby (the one transported by 'us', the brigade), 'our' infusion machines, 'our' incubator (as opposed to the one of the maternity hospital). In this way, I also symbolically included myself in the group of the brigade, thus counting myself among the 'participants'.

Subsequently, the trust and 'inclusive' attitude demonstrated by the intensive care staff raised questions of how to write about their work in a way that would not undermine this trust or offend anyone. There was also the question of how not to incur the wrath of colleagues against the physician co-author who made our study possible by allowing us into the field and who actually made sure that the team members were well disposed to social science scholars and trusted us a priori. It seems to me, notwithstanding these anxieties, that the attempt not to criticise but to find interpretations and anthropological explanations for the behaviour and statements of our informants in the methodology of thick description (Geertz 2008) avoids this potential threat even in the case of sensitised material.

The anthropologist influences the field by their presence, disturbing and disquieting the environment under study. I had to consider how my presence influenced the practices of doctors and nurses and to what extent their behaviour during their work routine became a performance that was played out in front of the researcher. I could envision my impact to some extent: for example, a nurse might talk more actively to a child or emphasise the attention she pays to a mother, a doctor might experience more anxiety in a difficult situation knowing that she or he is being observed. At the same time, it seems to me that the frame of urgency and deep involvement of the participants in the activity minimised these 'distortions', which are certainly usually informative for the researcher, in this field.

At the same time, any field that involves a certain degree of immersion does not pass without a trace for the anthropologist. The anthropologist does not simply observe what happens to her or his informants, but experiences emotions and feelings (cf. Capurro 2021 on the emotional work of the researcher during a field in a paediatric hospital). These emotions and feelings, on the one hand, can be informative for him – when a participant observer experiences something, it is a reason to reflect and ask how it is for others, what they feel. At the same time, in a field where the observer is not a full participant and does not share professional affiliation and professional skills (including emotional skills) with the informants, such self-observation as a data-gathering tool cannot be applied directly. In contrast to my previous research experience, here I was aware that medical detachment, which is formed during the professional socialisation of the medical professional, transforms the physician's optics and affects their experiences – in ways that do not obviously coincide with my lay view (for a discussion of the professional socialisation of the medical professional, including in relation to the formation of medical detachment, see the classic work of Becker et al. 1961). Nevertheless, I can suggest that my anxiety about the baby's condition, or my melting feeling at its animated appearance, or my sympathy for his mother, or my irritation at the indifference of the maternity hospital staff, all became, to some extent, our shared experiences with the medical participants.

The anthropologist, as a professional who is trained to behave in a certain way in the field, to switch registers of communication, vary their behaviour, and present different facets of their identity, nevertheless has that human part that they cannot change – for example, gender, age, ethnicity, social status. In some cases, this determines which fragments of the reality under study are available to the anthropologist: so perhaps the fact that I am a fairly young woman made my presence in a field related to motherhood less visible and more accountable. Perhaps the presence of an older male researcher, occupied with nothing, in a maternity ward would have raised more questions. At the same time, it is likely that the way we entered the field (a joint project with a doctor with high hierarchical and symbolic status in the community under study) would have helped to more or less alleviate these issues.

However, it is equally important to me that my 'built-in' characteristics have entered into a certain interaction with the sensitivity of the field and partly determined the extent of my participation in fieldwork. I first came to the field at the age of 34 and returned at 38, with no children of my own, but with reproductive plans in mind. Observing babies who were profoundly premature or born with certain pathologies, stories of mothers who had their uteruses removed after delivery, remarks by medical staff like 'Mom is forty, it is clear why [something is wrong with the baby]', or heartfelt stories from doctors about their encounters with the deaths of their baby-patients – all that evoked more than just empathy for me. Despite my mastery of professional (anthropological, in my case) techniques of detachment, I found it difficult not to project these stories onto my own possible or impossible motherhood or to reflect on my own decisions in this regard. In addition, in previous research projects, as I have already written, I have studied disabled childhood: on the one hand, the institutional context of specialised orphanages (Klepikova 2017), and on the other hand, parental experiences in families with children with disabilities (Klepikova 2019). Many of the children I had observed before in previous projects had also gone through infant resuscitation, and I was well aware of both the dehumanising experience of institutionalisation for such children and the hardships of parents raising a child with disabilities in Russia. I could not get rid of the thought that I could imagine the future of the infants I encountered during my fieldwork in case of an insufficiently favourable treatment outcome. Perhaps if my background had been different, I would have perceived the observation and interview materials in a less personalised manner, and this would have allowed me to conduct fieldwork (in particular, field trips as a participant observer) more intensively. But what I had to do was to consciously place restrictions on myself in this project, trying to regulate my own emotional state. I would like to point out that our physician interlocutors shared similar experiences: the impact of their work on their own reproductive plans and strategies, fears about childbirth and the delivery process among their relatives. They also complained that the fact that they did not see 'healthy' children, similar to me in my research projects, led to a certain kind of professional deformation. In a way, the only difference between me and our interviewees here was that I could 'leave the field' and they had to continue their work.

No less important than my key emotion in the field was the admiration from observing this work: the coordinated actions of the team physicians and medical nurses, the complex intellectual search for the right therapeutic solutions, the precise, highly professional reactions in emergency situations – and secretly, I envied their 'way of life' and the high importance of their mission. I see my mission in this book as, among other things, sharing how complex – physically, emotionally, bureaucratically and organisationally – their work is. Our research is, for me, the first experience of such a close interdisciplinary collaboration between medical and social sciences, in which, on the one hand, the medical community under study is given a powerful voice and, on the other, the perspective of the medical profession enriches the sociological and anthropological view.

Co-author Anastasia: Sociologist

Fieldwork in the sphere of neonatal resuscitation is not my first experience of ethnographic work in medical organisations, nor even my first experience of observing medical interactions with newborn patients and the work of paediatric resuscitators. Nevertheless, even though there are nosological (obstetrics and neonatology) and organisational (maternity hospitals) similarities between some of the empirical fields in which I have worked, each of them is defined by a unique configuration of how exactly access was granted to it, how the dynamics of my research position developed in the process, and the relationships within the research team (Novkunskaya et al. 2021). Taking the opportunity to speak here as an individual research unit, I will attempt to identify those methodological, ethical and disciplinary features of this research that were unexpected and most significant to me both professionally and personally.

In a previous study, I also worked in a research team of three colleagues (sociologists) with whom we conducted an institutional ethnography of a large maternity hospital. In that project, we also reflected upon the differences in our positions in the field and the influence of different social statuses (gender, age, professional position) on how research participants interacted with us. In particular, we discussed how repeatedly the researcher's position became negotiable and somewhat reassembled to fit both our own characteristics and the research objectives and circumstances of a particular interaction. We have also described how the position of 'insider' or 'outsider' in the field is not an unconditional reality, but rather a dynamically shifting relationship with the research participants.

Entering the field in the case of the current research seemed to be much more straightforward and linear, since one of the members of the research team (the co-author-physician) is also one of the key participants in the interactions being studied. However, the relatively simple entry into the field (which I personally initially perceived as research luck and a rare chance) did not remove all the dilemmas of my research position on the outsider-insider spectrum and even gave birth to new ones. On the one hand, our colleague, who was both part of the research team and part of the field under study, provided almost unlimited access to very different situations of interaction that, without such a resource, we would never have been able to observe. Intensive care units are quite closed (both formally and symbolically) loci, not only for 'outsiders' in relation to the medical field but sometimes even for the patient's relatives.

The guarantee of such access for us (sociologist and anthropologist) was both the rather high formal status of our colleague, as he became the head of the resuscitation and consultative service in 2022, and his informal symbolic capital – his professional experience and expertise were unequivocally recognised by almost all the doctors and nurses we met during our fieldwork. These statuses were undoubtedly a key resource for successful integration into the field and collection of a large amount of empirical data, but at the same time, they created additional risks (primarily reputational) and additional responsibility for us as social scholars.

Thus, even in situations where I was physically alone and observed as an independent researcher, I was presented and perceived by field participants primarily as Artemiy's (co-author-physician) colleague:

> [the intensive care transportation team and I are in the neonatal intensive care unit of a maternity hospital]. A male doctor (I later found out that he was the head of pediatric intensive care at maternity hospital X) points at me and addresses me as if to everyone: 'Who is this? standing here with a phone [I was recording notes on it for my field diary], the one who doesn't work!'.
>
> The intensive care transportation team doctor replies, 'That's ours, we need her, all additional questions address to Artemiy! [co-author doctor]'.
>
> The local female doctor also jokingly, addressing the superintendent: 'Why are you yelling? Hire her!'. The intensive care doctor replies something like, 'we need her ourselves!', The male doctor laughs, winks at me and walks away. (Observation diary, July 2023)

In our book, we study, among other things, the phenomenon of the 'extended patient', when the parents of the newborn are included in multiple medical communications as a social extension of the newborn. Similarly, I could say that I felt part of the 'extended researcher' when I, like the newborn patients, was hardly an independent subject, but a kind of extension of Artemiy's professional project. The more frightening thing was to 'screw up' the field – even the slightest conflict could lead not only to my own reputational and research losses but could bring harm to our dear colleague.

Other features of such a fieldwork position, in which it is not always possible to separate oneself as an individual researcher from the research team and in which a member of the research collective is very deeply integrated into the field, were professional tensions and conflicts of interest that created both ethical and methodological difficulties. For example, we did not immediately agree amongst ourselves whether to conduct focus groups on emotional work with nurses (rather than just physicians). When we did, there was a question of how to recruit participants, as some nursing staff may have perceived our physician colleague as a controlling authority. Solutions to these ethical and methodological difficulties were to enlist the help of our colleagues who did not have a professional relationship with Artemiy to recruit the informants and to conduct the focus group itself with nursing staff without his participation.

The differences in our professional (academia and practical health care) and disciplinary (neonatology, anthropology, sociology) positions were also evident at times in our working negotiations outside the field: in discussions about how and what data we wanted to collect, how we should analyse the data already collected, and even in some interpretations of the same observations. The most valuable for me, both personally and professionally, was the synchronisation of our views and positions and the very possibility of writing in all other parts of the book from our common research voice.

Research Design

We deliberately began the methodological chapter of our book with the personal voicing of the perspective of each of the researchers. By doing so, we not only immediately articulate the ethical and epistemological limitations of our research design and methodology but also reveal that research reflection, the search for working (interdisciplinary) solutions for collecting and analysing empirical data, and the development of a common language (since the book is written from our collective authorial 'we') have been as important an outcome of our work as the analytical conclusions which we have drawn. So, here we switch back into the writing mode of a cohesive author team and present the key features of our research design so that the reader can evaluate the validity, reliability and consistency of our data and the results of their analysis.

Crucial to the study design is the fact that our research focus is on the multiple social perspectives and contexts that define the position and entities of the newborn patient in the medical community and health care settings. We aim to show that patients with similar characteristics and medical status who are in the same organisational contexts actually manifest different 'selves': physical and medical, social, economic and even political. At the same time, when dealing with a patient 'without a personal biography' (e.g., a newborn and especially a patient born prematurely), and in some cases – 'without a future' (since some of them have very high risks of unfavourable outcomes), our study points to universal mechanisms of constructing the medical position of the 'patient' that depend on the institutional context in which she or he is located. These research objectives determined the methodological tools we have chosen.

The study was carried out with the application of a qualitative methodology and involved the use of several methods for data collection and analysis:

1. Analysis of documents relevant to the history of neonatal service in the study region and neonatal care in Russia; analysis of legal documents defining the status of a newborn, the procedure for neonatal care and professional standards for the work of specialists in this profile. This method was applied to investigate and describe the historical, organisational and legal background of the study (for more details, see appendix 6).
2. In order to deepen the data on the history and some organisational features of neonatology in the region of study, we conducted a series of expert interviews with healthcare managers and administrators, as well as with those professionals who pioneered the organisation of neonatal care in the city. A guide for expert semi-structured interviews was elaborated by the research team (for more details, see appendix 1), all the members of the research team participated in this data collection.
3. The dataset consisted of interviews with the heads of neonatal pathology departments of paediatric hospitals, interview with the chief freelance specialist in the field of neonatology, interview with the deputy chief physician for administrative and expert work of a paediatric hospital, interview with the head of the palliative home care supply department, interview with the head of the neonatal intensive care department of a paediatric hospital (one of the first in the region), and two interviews with physician consultants of the transport service, who stood at the origins of the opening of the service (for more details on this data, see appendix 3).
4. A series of semi-structured interviews with doctors and nurses providing resuscitation and neonatal care (doctors and nurses of paediatric hospitals; doctors and nurses providing emergency and consultative care; doctors and nurses of maternity hospitals). This method was

among the first applied to the study as it enabled learning in more detail the health professionals' perspective on the most challenging and sensitive issues faced in their medical practice. All the interviews were conducted by Artemiy Minakov in the years 2019–2021 (for more details, see appendix 3).

5. The core empirical data comprising our study is the series of self-observations, conducted by Artemiy Minakov in the course of his own work as a RAC (transport intensive care) physician. The dataset consists of 33 on-call visits (116 pages of diary entries, for more details, see appendix 4). Diary records were kept with varying regularity over three years. Outside the observation period, some events that seemed important for one reason or another were also recorded in the form of field notes. The data collection initially did not pursue the goal of publication, nor did it have a clear formulation of the object and subject of the research, but all the data were read and discussed by all the members of the research team and then inspired the whole study to be conducted.
6. In order to immerse ourselves (anthropologist and sociologist) into the field of study, to learn more about the daily routine and communicative practices of health professionals providing neonatal care, we decided to conduct additional (to the self-observations by Artemiy) ethnographic observations of the work of the medical staff of the transport intensive care service, maternity hospitals, and the intensive care unit of the paediatric hospital. Thus, in 2023, Anna and Anastasia conducted seven observations, overall lasting for 61 hours (75 pages of diary entries, for more details, see appendix 4).
7. While conducting ethnographic observations, we noticed that the emotional work of doctors and nurses dealing with newborn patients comprised an important (although not always recognised and visible) dimension of their work. Thus, we decided to address the emotional work of health professionals in particular. Based on the methodological discussions (Smithson 2000; Acocella, 2011), the method of focus groups was selected to learn more about the emotional labour of health practitioners, which was substantiated by three main arguments. Firstly, we recognise that emotional work is a sensitive issue and opted for collective discussion as the one providing more comfortable and supportive conditions for our research participants. Secondly, we had a hypothesis that organisational norms and cultures shape considerably the way emotions are experienced and articulated (for more details see chapter 4), and thus, wanted to compare different sectors of neonatal care (maternity hospitals, RAC, paediatric hospitals) as well as different professional groups (doctors and nurses). The data collected in the

frame of focus groups allowed us to implement this comparison in a more systematic way. And thirdly, focus groups as a method enable researchers to collect not only narrative data but also the one on the dynamics of the group discussion. In this way, we supposed that the collective reactions to our questions would allow us to detect the most sensitive and triggering topics and themes (related to emotional labour) for the groups under study.

To conduct focus groups we elaborated a topic-guide (for more details see appendix 2), and invited for participation representatives of the following professional groups:

1. Neonatal nurse practitioners, working in RAC and maternity hospitals
2. Neonatal nurses, working in the neonatal intensive care unit of a paediatric hospital
3. Physicians, working in the neonatal intensive care unit of a paediatric hospital
4. Physicians working in the neonatal intensive care units of maternity hospitals
5. Physicians working in the RAC (transport intensive care service). (For more details on this data, see appendix 5.)

Overall, the field study and data collection took place intermittently from the second half of 2019 through November 2023. The method of selection of research participants was as follows: The target group during interviews and focus groups with doctors and nurses was the medical staff providing neonatal and resuscitation care to newborns during the study period. Recruitment of informants was essentially done through the social networks of one of the researchers, which largely determined the research strategy during the material collection phase.

Expert interviews with the medical professionals who pioneered the organisation of neonatal care became a unique case sample; we focused on currently available informants who have worked in the study region since the 1970s.

DATA ANALYSIS

The first stage of data analysis was the transcription of interviews and focus group audio recordings verbatim. All personal data was then colour-tagged for subsequent anonymisation. In the case of diary entries, the researchers took notes as detailed as possible during the observation and then fleshed out details after leaving the field on the very same day.

All researchers reread all the textual data in a continuous manner and then discussed key empirical plots. This stage of data analysis can be referred to as a method of 'meaning condensation' (Kvale 2003), that is, the extracting and summarising of emerging meaning units. In most cases, such meaning units were noted in the format of intra-textual comments by all the researchers.

The key stage of data analysis was a combination of deductive and inductive coding (Flick 2009), depending on the goals of each of the empirical chapters. For the first empirical chapter (see chapter 3, 'Nothing personal') an open-coding method was used to detect the emic terms (or 'labels') used in interactions between health professionals and patients ('boy', 'girl', 'kyzy-myzy', 'illigals', 'foetus', '600 g', etc.). We then grouped these codes into more general codes ('gender labels, ethnic labels, professional communication, personal names', etc.) and further categorised them into more abstract and analytical classifications, consisting of 'medical labels' and 'social labels'.

For the second empirical chapter (see chapter 4) we inductively conducted a thematic analysis, analysing what themes, related to the emotional dimension of professional work in neonatal care emerged in our field notes, informants' narratives, or focus group discussions. This step, in particular, highlighted key issues related to the forms of emotional labour of medical professionals. The structure of chapter 4 correlates with the key themes found, springing from the empirical data. For the third empirical chapter (chapter 5) we analysed the empirical data mostly deductively, focusing on those data fragments which corresponded to the pre-identified categories of bureaucracy, politics, legal issues, resources and material infrastructures. In particular, we selected data that described the documentary, organisational, political, or infrastructural features of neonatal care.

ETHICAL DILEMMAS OF THE RESEARCH

'The birth of the patient' project was supported by the Associate Professorship on Qualitative Health Research (based at the European University at Saint-Petersburg) and received ethical approval from the St. Petersburg Association of Sociologists. Nevertheless, in the process of implementing the project data collection and analysis, many ethical questions and dilemmas arose, which we additionally had to think of, reflect on and solve. One of the key ethical difficulties of our research was the extreme sensitivity of the field under study. In the course of our work, conducting observations, interviews and focus groups, we were constantly confronted with the pain, suffering and emotional fatigue of our research participants. This required methodological care and extra sensitivity not to reinforce the vulnerabilities and challenges already existing in this field.

This sensitivity also caused emotional difficulties for the researchers themselves. We were not always able to show the degree of engagement and empathy with observed events. One solution to this ethical dilemma was to conduct focus groups on the emotional labour of doctors and nurses working in the field. This method, besides collecting empirical data, also addressed the issue of increasing the visibility of the sensitive experiences, suffering and hard work of the medical professionals under study. The focus group situation appeared to be also an opportunity to talk about troubling feelings and experiences and to share difficult experiences in a safe environment. In this way, the focus group situation can be seen as a kind of quasi-psychotherapy. Of course, we do not have the necessary expertise for this, and we did not set any therapeutic goals for this method application, but we received, among other things, grateful feedback for the fact that colleagues could share their experiences in such a format. Thus, we follow the ethical principle of reciprocity and hope that our research will enhance the visibility of the emotional work done by health providers. In addition to the methodology applied, the very style of the manuscript in the empirical part reflects our intention to give voice to our interlocutors. Partly for this reason, the manuscript contains quite lengthy quotations. That is a deliberate solution, as we wanted to give voice and symbolic space to our interlocutors in the text, as well as to problematise the ethnographic data collection in the very sensitive field of research.

In addition, during our fieldwork, we tried not to disturb our research participants as much as possible. In the process of collecting interviews and making arrangements to meet with the researchers, the project participants drew on the principles of convenience for and availability of the informants themselves. Typically, interviews took place at the informant's workplace, during or after their duty hours, at a time when the informant had the opportunity to give the researchers time. A few focus groups took place in the office of one of the researchers at the university, which was also geographically convenient for all participants. During the interview process, our guide was adjusted to the amount of time our interlocutors were willing to give us. During the communication of the research, we followed etiquette and ethical norms, such as polite and correct treatment of informants; informing them about the purpose of the research and the professional status of its performers; sensitivity to the sensory experience and attention to the emotions of informants. Informants were told at the beginning of the interview that they had the right to refuse to answer any of the questions. Informants had the right to refuse to participate in the study at any stage.

At the same time, the suffering and pain of patients (including 'extended patients', for more details on the emotional experiences of women in cases of perinatal losses, see Litvina, 2022) remained less disclosed in our project. This was both a deliberate methodological and ethical decision by our research team, as we did not include patients directly in the focus of our research, focusing on the actions, the communications of medical professionals and the organisational social contexts in which they work. Thus, while studying patients and their trajectories, we actually left them faded into the background, as we did not want to unintentionally traumatise them, to stress them, or to reinforce the state of uncertainty in which they already were for the most part of being in the field under study.

Another ethical difficulty of our project is related to ensuring the conditions of anonymity of participation. Our project has a number of regional features that make it virtually impossible to anonymise the city. Moreover, the affiliation of one of the researchers, and the fact that he was conducting a participatory observation, did not allow for complete anonymity of the whole field of study. Nevertheless, we have taken all possible steps to provide anonymity for all the other research participants at all stages of the project. The anonymity of participation is ensured by following strict rules for transcribing audio recordings of interviews, as informants were assigned pseudonyms at the transcription stage. In the instructions for transcribers, we have also noted the need to strictly respect the confidentiality of information. At the stage of manuscript preparation, some additional measures providing anonymity have been taken. In the text, we do not mention personal names or other personal details, we also do not mention the names of the medical organisations in which our research participants worked. The pseudonyms are used inconsistently across the manuscript (the very same research participant can have different pseudonyms in different chapters). We also omit mentioning any official and full job titles, as well as the exact ages and other personal details of our research participants.

Finally, the third ethical dilemma of our research is related to the complex position (or rather positions) of the researchers in the field. On the one hand, Artemiy's immersion in all the professional interactions in the neonatal care of the region ensured that we all were able to enter it, giving us access to collect various empirical data. On the other hand, this required additional care and reflexivity in maintaining some analytical distance between practical engagement and research. Thus, with their different disciplinary backgrounds, all three members of the research team dealt with this ethical challenge in different ways and answered for themselves how to maintain a balance of participation and non-participation, involvement and non-involvement, empathy and some research detachment.

Participant observations were conducted in the project by several researchers with different levels of inclusion, which ensures the triangulation of methods and data. On the one hand, the participant observations were conducted by the co-author-physician as part of his professional (neonatal intensive care physician) and job (head of department) responsibilities. The object of observation is the work of the resuscitation team and the decisions made by the neonatal service. At the same time, all study participants were warned about the study. On the other hand, non-participant observations were conducted by co-authors, a sociologist and an anthropologist, who are 'external' observers to the transport intensive care service. Their research status and research aims were also communicated to the participants. The focus of observation may also include the work of maternity hospital staff, their interaction with newborns and medical decisions in which they are involved. In such cases, researchers additionally inform maternity hospital staff about the study (including the participation of 'external' observers), its goals and objectives.

The study was conducted under epidemiologically and politically unfavourable conditions (COVID-19 pandemic, war in Ukraine), but the topic and objectives of the study do not directly relate to these circumstances, although material relating to the pandemic situation and military conditions inevitably made its way into our data. The researchers sought to observe both ethical and epidemiologic precautions to avoid increasing the vulnerabilities and potential risks of study participants.

LIST OF APPENDICES

Appendix 1: Guide for Expert and Biographical Interviews with Medical Professionals Involved in the Institutionalization of Neonatology Since the Late 1970s
Appendix 2: Guide for a Focus Group with Physicians and Nurses in the Neonatology Service
Appendix 3: List of Informants and Description of Interviews
Appendix 4: List of Observations
Appendix 5: List and Description of Focus Groups
Appendix 6: List of Archival Documents

Chapter 3

Nothing Personal

INTRODUCTION

This chapter addresses the phenomenon of medicalisation in an organisational context, applying conceptual tools of the interactionist perspective, labelling theory in particular. Focusing on the interactions of medical professionals with each other and with the patients, including their extended version (parents of a newborn – for further discussion of the concept of extended patient, see chapter 4), we conceptualise medicalisation as a continuum in which constant switching of communicative registries takes place. We analyse how medicalisation in multiple organisational contexts is enacted in different ways and how differently it shapes the processes of objectification of a patient versus endowing him or her with agency. We analyse the medical and social categories (labels) used by health professionals to categorise newborn patients as reflecting different organisational contexts, on the one hand, and shaping the patients' trajectories on the other.

'The Social System' by Talcott Parsons claims that the sick role turns out to be leading for a sick person, while other social statuses fade into the background in the context of a medical appointment or hospitalisation (Parsons 1951a, b). Being a patient in a hospital, a person is deprived of his or her ordinary social roles. Once anthropologist Robert Murphy entered the hospital as a patient, he understood that gender, age and social position played only a small role in his institutionalised interactions with medical professionals, because the hospital routine was indifferent to those statuses (Murphy 1987, 19–22). At the same time, marketisation changes interactions between a doctor and a patient: for example, researchers report that 'patients' become more and more agentic, for their role is redefined, they are treated like 'clients' (service recipients), and their interaction with medical institutions and healthcare in general depends on their access to material, social and symbolic resources (Temkina 2017). The political system plays an important role in the context of such interactions, since certain social policies give additional meaning to the status of the patient (we will discuss this in more detail in chapter 5). Such measures form certain rules of interaction in organisational conditions and affect the way medical staff treat a patient, who is a newborn with pathologies in our particular case.

Any patient receiving medical care interacts with many specialists, each of whom forms his or her own 'patient image', using convenient and appropriate labels. Not all of them can be unambiguously deciphered outside of a specific organisational context, and most of these labels refer to 'emic' categories, that is, to the terms that the community under study uses to classify the phenomena of the surrounding world. These terms can often be incomprehensible and seem ambiguous to ordinary people or, to some extent, even unethical. However, within a certain professional environment, they help to determine the patient's condition most accurately, which includes him or her in everyday work in a convenient and predictable way.

We propose to use the term 'a label' as a characteristic, which helps professionals form their idea of a newborn, expressing it in the process of their interprofessional communication through special designations (emic terms) or social references (gender and name). Analysing those labels, we reconstruct the logic of various organisational contexts, as well as trace the effect of one or another label on the patient's treatment trajectory. At the same time, the newborn patient remains passive in accepting the labels offered to him or her by medical specialists and in following the social norms expected from this role. As for an adult patient in Parsons' interpretation, the sick role becomes the leading one for the newborn patient, but the difference from his concept is that at this stage of life of the baby all other roles and communicative intentions are ascribed to him or her by the adults.

MEDICALISATION AND LABELLING PROCESS

Medicalisation as a social phenomenon and as a concept in the social sciences has been studied for more than half a century. The growing importance and influence of medicine as a social institution in post-industrial societies resulted in critical attempts to comprehend social processes through the category of medicalisation. As soon as the first conceptualisations of this phenomenon began, medicalisation researchers paid their attention to historical and macro-social changes in society's attitudes towards medicine, health and treatment. According to Irwin Zola, one of the first sociologists who developed the concept of medicalisation, 'Health has turned from a simple means of achieving good into the main good and goal of human existence', while medicine itself has turned into 'an institution of social control' (Zola 1972; see also Illich 1976; Mikhel 2011, 256).

Research on the phenomenon of medicalisation has gone through several stages and has addressed the study of different social contexts and human experiences. Summarising the key ways in which the concept is conceptualised in social research, two main definitions of medicalisation can be given. This is, firstly, the increasing power of medical institutions in society, whose powers go beyond the treatment and prevention of diseases and cover the functions of social control, for example, the required narcologist and psychiatrist examinations for admission to work as an anaesthesiologist on a mobile anaesthesia team. And secondly, it is the redefinition of social phenomena in medical categories and the interpretation of social problems as pathological, that is, related to the medical field (Mikhel 2009, 293; Conrad 1992). For example, even a physiologically normal pregnancy is now subject to close monitoring and examination, and childbirths outside a medical institution may be considered semi-illegal (Temkina et al. 2022). In Russia, the law does not allow a midwife, gynaecologist, or other health practitioner to assist with home births. Medical professionals who agree to provide maternity are at risk of criminal prosecution, although parents of a newborn can opt to give birth in any place and refuse facility-based services.

This chapter focuses on the definition or interpretation of an infant born with pathologies from the point of view of medical categories and within the framework of medical discourse. We propose here to nuance the understanding of de/medicalisation and study it not only as a historical process of increasing control by medical institutions and redefining social phenomena in medical categories, but also as a certain register of communication taking place in a medical context. Our analytical objectives here are to study the mechanisms of de/medicalisation as a process of redefining communication and social relations in medical categories, associated with the process of patient objectification at the microlevel of social interaction. First, this way of conceptualising helps to consider the relativity of medicalisation and its dependence on different organisational contexts. Secondly, addressing the linguistic and communicative aspects of this phenomenon, we aim to show how, in a highly medicalised context, communication produces a social subject, and how, even in such conditions, the interaction with the patient can be demedicalised. Thus, we aim to contribute to the classic social science and humanities discussion of medicalisation by applying this category to analyse the microlevel of social interaction.

This work focuses on the production of statuses in medical interactions; therefore, it approaches the object of study within an interactionist perspective and relies on the conceptual model of labels (labelling theory) in the analysis of medicalisation. The concept of labelling in its various variants (Becker 1963; Goffman 1961; Goffman 1963; Lemert 1951; Rosenhan 1973) is an attempt to explain how society labels a particular behaviour as deviant, and how these labels determine the individual's further trajectory within social institutions. According to the labelling theory, a medical context implies that a diagnosis made to a patient is a sort of interface, which further mediates and determines the interaction of medical personnel with him or her. Other characteristics of the patient and attempts to construct his or her identity in a different way fade into the background. This work leaves aside aspects related to the construction of deviance; it studies the functioning of the labels that newborns acquire during medical communication and the ways of reference used by medical professionals. To what extent do these labels and references, being related to a specific organisational context, determine an infant's trajectory within and between medical institutions?

Previous researchers have shown that healthcare practitioners tend to assign the 'social case' label to patients whose social problems are more pressing than the medical ones (see, for example, Wamsiedel 2016). However, the case under study is extreme in terms of the degree of medicalisation – it considers not just a child, but a newborn with severe pathologies, who, as a rule, is in a state of sedation and vitally depends on life-support equipment. Consequently, even the usual ways to express himself or herself, characteristic of infants (e.g., crying, moving), are not available to them. In addition, a significant part of the time they are alienated from their parents, who usually make a significant contribution to the creation of his or her identity.

Although not all interactions are associated with the provision of emergency and technological care in some sectors of the field under study (e.g., in the case of children born without health problems), we focus on those cases that suggest an already diagnosed medical pathology or suspicion of it. By default, such interactions are highly medicalised, but the empirical evidence presented in the next section allows them to be analysed as a more complex spectrum of social relationships. Thus, the focus of attention is largely not medicalisation per se, but the opposite, demedicalising trends that exist in this highly medicalised field.

In this chapter, we study the way of attaching different professional 'labels' to the same newborn patient, depending on what stage of observation and treatment he or she is at and what institution he or she is in, as well as the manner in which these labels are used by medical professionals in their daily work practices. Using the multiplicity of these medical and non-medical terms, we suggest analysing the formation of different understandings of the patient in different organisational contexts, as well as reflecting this understanding in different practices of medical professionals.

THE BIRTH OF A PATIENT

A newborn with pathologies is left alone with the medical system; there, he or she is forced to alienate himself or herself from his or her parents and integrate into established practices of treatment and care. His or her emotional reactions are perceived by the medical staff primarily as indicators of physiological states rather than social action, although, as will be shown later, there are different approaches in different groups of health personnel in this regard. This does not exclude the subjective interaction of medical workers with a patient, but it can lead to conflict in the case when the professional view of the patient fades into the background:

> While we were setting up the equipment, the child burst into tears, and nurse Sasha asked, 'Is this *a boy*?' The nurse at the hospital said yes. Then Sasha began to intensively stroke his hand saying, '*boys* love being pitied'. (Diary of participant observations, maternity hospital, October 2020)

On the one hand, this kind of nurse's reaction to crying shows that she perceives him not only as a patient, but also as a person, attributing widespread gender stereotypes to him. On the other hand, such a reaction can be regarded by doctors as unprofessional, as it leads away from the search for the causes of the child's anxiety, whether it is a physiological or pathological process (hunger, pain, etc.). It is worth comparing the description of the professional development of a doctor, which implies a refusal to understand what is happening with patients in categories of common sense, in the classic work of Howard Becker and colleagues (Becker et al. 1961). During our fieldwork, we could clearly observe the differences in interactions with patients depending on the severity of their state:

> Doctor Elena enters the ward and starts calling the baby Musik. In general, the baby seems to be quite stable, pink (they discuss his 'good' colour) and even opens his eyes – 'his eyes have opened'. So he immediately gets a lot of compliments like 'so good' and '*fighter*'. All this is said in a reassuring tone. The boy is the second of twins, but the girl is not on the vent, as the head of the department says when asked about it by Elena. '*Girls are fighters!*' says Elena. (Diary of participant observations, maternity hospital, July 2023)
>
> Already no one coddles the baby much, because he is in more severe condition, more complicated and unclear, requires more interventions, 'tubes' – less normal functioning. 'Pretty' the same health practitioners say of another baby who is lying without [oxygen supply] tubes. The nurse calls a second baby good-looking, redhead 'big-eared' – perhaps he has bigger ears, and will be

> transported by another team. He's just kind of jaundiced. (Diary of participant observations, maternity hospital, July 2023)

Despite the fact that a newborn is surrounded by medical professionals from the moment of birth, it would be erroneous to say that his or her development as a patient is associated only with biological and pathological processes; some factors that are not directly related to the disease play a significant role in the process of interaction between medical professionals and the child. Habitual attributes that are significant for communication outside the medical context, such as gender, name, or related social statuses, do not disappear but go to the periphery, and statuses specific to the medical environment take their dominant place. The number of such statuses varies and depends on the severity of his or her condition, the social status of his or her parents, and the organisational conditions of the institution in which he or she receives treatment.

> A nurse comes in and asks: 'Well, what is waiting for us?' doctor Lena says with indignation: '600 g in the N maternity hospital, born after breech presentation and had no therapy except for Curosurf'. Lena continues: his butt and legs are probably bruised, he should be anesthetised, anaesthesia reduces blood pressure, so additional drugs [are needed] . . . (Diary of participant observations, children's hospital RAC, July 2023)

In this quote, we observe how a doctor, upon hearing medical data (labels) including the weight of a newborn, the institution in which he or she was born, and the circumstances of birth, immediately identifies one of the possible treatment options. This clearly demonstrates how labels – in this case, markers of a certain condition, even before the patient is examined – set a certain predisposition to treatment. In addition to the medical indicators themselves, such a predisposition to treatment is also shaped by the status of the maternity care institution in which a patient was born – whether it has a 'good reputation' among professionals or not. This status is partly influenced by the way the facility is funded – whether it is private or state-funded. The development of the commercial sector in healthcare also changes the rules of interaction with a patient, which becomes especially noticeable when compared to the public one.

> Ulyana (the RAC doctor) regrets and resents that there are a lot of money and resources spent on a non-viable child. Secondly, she condemns private medicine, in which, for whatever purpose, [doctors] dissuaded the mum from having an abortion. In general, when women choose private maternity hospitals – they care about themselves! And not about the baby. Why not to be patient just for

three days, but then you are guaranteed to receive high-quality care and free of charge. If something is wrong with a baby, any additional service is to be paid in a private maternity hospital, any analysis. And the very same procedures will be for free in any state-funded [maternity hospital]. And in a private no one will tell the truth! They will say, 'Everything will be fine, the child will go to school!' even when there are clearly no chances. (Diary of participant observations, intensive care ambulance RAC, June 2023)

This narrative of a doctor working in the public healthcare sector demonstrates a clearly paternalistic approach to the treatment process, which contrasts the requirement of comfort with quality of care. As previous studies (Temkina et al. 2022) have shown, women do indeed often choose the private health sector because of greater comfort. However, in addition to the comfort conditions for labour and postnatal stay, they also often pay for a more personalised approach and the opportunity to experience more agency as patients. Without clinical expertise, patients are often unable to assess the safety and adequacy of the care they receive. At the same time, we see that their expectations for more comfort and personification of care create additional tension for doctors and nurses, who elaborate an additional social label for patients born in the commercial sector. We will particularly address the effects of such social labels on patients' trajectories in more detail in the next section.

SOCIAL REFERENCES IN DIFFERENT ORGANISATIONAL CONTEXTS

A child's name and gender are important identifiers of a newborn that are among the first to emerge, often before birth. The name and affectionate and playful nicknames are the references that parents and relatives use in everyday life in the process of interacting with the child from the moment of birth, while gender is the basic cultural classification category, which is formalised and emphasised by special means and frames social interactions (Ridgeway 2009).

In a medical context, a child's last name, date of birth, gender and anthropometrics are recorded on a tag, with which the child moves within and between organisations. At the same time, the frequency of using the surname as an identifier varies depending on the sector of neonatal care. Thus, in the transit sector, where interaction with a child is intense but short, the patient's surname is part of the medical documentation and rarely comes up in the communication process. This can be seen in the formal resuscitation and advisory centre (RAC) morning conferences, where doctors report on the work done or discuss individual clinical cases, and informal conversations between doctors during the shift transfer period. 'A child of 2,600 g was transferred, on the third day with a diagnosis of SDR,' says a typical report of a RAC doctor; 'There, 600 g are waiting for you in the second maternity hospital, we have already visited him twice' is a common style of conversation between RAC doctors.

The use of certain references is also influenced by the professional socialisation of a particular doctor. If, for example, it took place in a different organisational context, the surname can also be used as an identifier:

> 'A girl named Suvorova was transferred (to the children's hospital) on the first day of her life, with a diagnosis . . .' says a report of a doctor working in a pediatric hospital and part-time at RAC. When one of RAC doctors began to use the child's surname during the report, RAC staff noticed that, commenting in an informal setting, 'Now you are like them . . .' which emphasised that 'ours' did not do that [use surnames].

Thus, differences in the use of certain labels reflect the informal boundaries that exist within the studied professional group, depending on the sector in which its activities are carried out. Indeed, the use of patients' surnames in the process of communication between RAC doctors seems redundant, since it does not provide information important for this sector. Therefore, when communicating with each other, RAC doctors often use the number of the maternity hospital and the leading syndrome or diagnosis when they want to talk about a patient:

> We have just taken the child to the hospital. In the hallway I ran into two ward nurses. They look unhappy and say, 'you filled us up with children today!' I answer that we still have one more *foetus* from the *XXth maternity hospital*. 'Yes, we know that. Alex [the responsible resuscitator] is already looking for an incubator for him'. (Diary of participant observations, children's hospital, December 2019)

As communication goes beyond their own sector, however, this way of transmitting information fails, since in hospitals doctors often have to interact with the patient's relatives and treat several patients with similar diagnoses/conditions at the same time. Therefore, they often use the child's last name and room number, rather than the name of the hospital in which he or she was born. When a doctor of the transfer team asks a conditional question, 'How is the aspirant[1] from the 14th maternity hospital, which I brought on Tuesday?', a counterquestion follows, 'What is his last name?'

Unlike the surname, which is entered into medical records immediately after birth and has a formal status (a 103/u-form), the first name does not appear in medical or other records until the birth certificate is received. In addition, not all parents have time to give a name to their child by the time of his or her birth (which is, in the context of the study, often premature). Doctors and nurses in many obstetric hospitals are interested in the name of a newborn and use it in communication with relatives or when interacting with the child. Sometimes parents themselves tell doctors about the name of a child:

> The child's mother was standing nearby and watching the nurses swaddling her child; at some point she turned to me and said, '*Hera* is a goddess (that was the child's name) . . . but how will she be fed? What are they going to do if she doesn't eat enough?' (Diary of participant observations, maternity hospital, November 2020)

According to the observation, nursing staff use names more often than other health practitioners in relation to newborns; usually, this occurs during physical interaction with the patients in the process of caring for them or feeding them. At the same time, the more severe a child's condition is, the less often he or she is called by name and the less subjectivity he or she is endowed with. So, a baby who breathes on his/her own, and whose condition has already been corrected, can be awarded the special attention of a nurse:

> A ward nurse is talking to babies, especially a lot with the one she likes, often calling him by name. 'You've got meconium in here, right?' she says exactly in the same tone as they say to babies, 'Did you poop?' She calls him 'bunny'. . . . While she is weighing him, she says, 'Do not even think about peeing'. When he is crying, she says, 'Good. You'll be bad. Maybe you'll go to your mother'? As she is putting on a pink vest on him, he soon begins to cry, she says, 'Are you crying because you are dressed in pink, you are upset?' She says that this is a good colour and that he is still a real big man, 'Give me your legs here'. (Diary of participant observations, maternity hospital, January 2020)

Doctors in intensive care units pay much less attention to the 'social' characteristics of a patient. For example, in communication with each other they rarely use the names and genders of their patients, replacing the words 'boy' or 'girl' with the more universal word 'child' or simply by default, using a masculine pronoun:

> There still seem to be 4 children in the ward, 'ours' is grey. . . . Soon I notice that ours is a girl, but everyone around calls her 'he'. (Diary of participant observations, maternity hospital, January 2020)

> The nurses start to change clothes, discover (even earlier, by the colour of the tag) that it is a girl. They say it is a girl to the doctor, who keeps calling a baby 'he'. She replies – hell with it! Meaning that gender doesn't matter. The nurses,

> especially the one who is not Lena, deal with it differently, already call a baby only 'she', while the doctor continues to use 'he', although produces some sort of minimal baby-talk. (Diary of participant observations, maternity hospital, November 2023)

While receiving care within the three sectors of neonatal care, a patient is embedded in different organisational settings and participates in interactions shaped by different professional tasks:

> We solve the problems of the first 24 hours of life, but also later on there . . . third, fourth, fifth, sixth [up to] 10 months of life. And the RAC doctor. . . . I also, in general, worked for quite a long time at the transport team, he solves his tasks. His task is to bring a person in a 'marketable appearance' (in good condition) to the ward. The task of a maternity hospital doctor, in my opinion, is primarily to identify borderline conditions and prevent fatal situations from developing. Therefore, of course, they are different. (An intensive care unit doctor, female, focus group materials, August 2023)

In most cases, children on artificial lung ventilation and receiving sedatives are admitted to the intensive care units of paediatric hospitals. Their activity is reduced, and interaction with them is limited to medical prescriptions. In relatively rare cases, when children in moderate or satisfactory condition are admitted to these departments, one can observe the interaction with such patients changing:

> The ward nurse immediately announced that the child, transferred to independent breathing, was called Ariadne. A heated discussion of unusual names immediately began. . . . Since the child still needed intensive observation, it was decided to transfer her to the intensive care unit. At the entrance, another ward nurse meets us and says, 'It's somehow indecent, there are even no nasal tubes (oxygen inhalation)'. At the desk, the doctor with a dissatisfied look says, 'Why did you bring her to us? You've separated the child from her mother! She'll be distracting me from work'! The nurses, examining the child, comment, 'They brought a funny chubby tot . . . she's pretty'. (Diary of participant observations, children's hospital, October 2020)

This example demonstrates the organisational differences between intensive care units in maternity and paediatric hospitals. Children who cannot continue treatment in the maternity hospital due to the severity of their condition are transferred to the intensive care units of paediatric hospitals. This naturally leads to the fact that 'serious' children (with severe pathologies or conditions) from all over the region are taken there, while children who do not need long-term respiratory support continue treatment in maternity hospitals. The transfer of such 'nonspecialised' patients for the purpose of short-term observation in the intensive care unit causes tenderness ('pretty', 'funny tot') or discontent ('she'll be distracting me'). Such reactions indicate an atypical situation since neonatal resuscitation patients rarely have the level of activity that implies personified interaction or using the name.

It is worth noting that the nurses of the intensive care units in paediatric hospitals often use the names of their patients when the patients are hospitalised for a long time. However, the arrival of a new (just-born) patient with a name is perceived by the medical staff as something unusual:

> At about 1 p.m. we handed over the child to the intensive care unit of the pediatric hospital. Leaving my desk, I said that the child's name was Arkady, and the nurse of the receiving hospital replied, 'Well, yes, maybe you can come up with a middle name[2] for him, too?!' (Diary of participant observations, children's hospital, October 2020)

Our materials show that different sectors have their own preferred references, which are used by professionals in identifying children (for more details on different patients' classifications, see chapter 4). These classifications comprise another set of medical labels:

> No, I have '*little ones*' – that's premature, asphyxiation and surgery [patients]. That's the division I have for myself. And '*relatively healthy*'. This is the nastiest contingent with the most difficult parents and probably the most difficult children to understand. Because they always don't realise what's hidden underneath their healthiness. (A doctor at the neonatal pathology department, female, focus group materials, September 2023)

> We also have such divisions as premature, surgical, cardiac and neurosurgical babies. . . . Well, you can go deeper. Bigger/smaller, heavier, minor [complications], with more difficult parents and less difficult parents. Still, you're paired up with the child and the mum. . . . Well, you immediately see both the mother and the child, and there is some kind of interpretation start. . . . It's purely on an emotional level. Some patients can be approached several times, and for others one time [to check on them] is enough. (A doctor at the neonatal pathology department, female, focus group materials, September 2023)

Neonatologists working in maternity hospitals, where the duration of a baby's stay is limited to a few hours or days, whose main task is to identify pathology, use more simple medical labels. For example, they describe their categorisation of newborns in focus groups as:

> 'Preterm, premature. Sick and healthy. Examined and unexamined', 'Probably understandable or obscure babies, in terms of initial treatment and diagnosis'.

Changes in familiar patterns cause reactions that emphasise the existing differences between the sectors: 'You are like them!', 'maybe you can come up with a middle name for him, too?!' At the same time, the labels themselves do not so much influence the formation of the patient's image or his or her treatment trajectory but rather reflect the structural and functional differences between the sectors. It is worth noting that the treatment trajectory means not only the patient's movement from one institution/department to another, which is determined by the institutional order and formally prescribed routing, but also a more nuanced organisation of this movement, in particular, the time spent on the transfer and the number of interactions involved. Thus, the influence of references and the set of labels on the treatment trajectory primarily mean the speed and efficiency of following the patient's route rather than its key points.

CONFLICT OF MEDICAL AND 'SOCIAL' STATUSES

Professional labels are often represented by emic categories that professionals use to communicate more effectively within the professional community. The labels convey information about a patient and can be combined into homogeneous groups. Some of them reflect the physical or pathological conditions of the patient, that is, 'foetus', 'stomach', 'asphyxiant', 'defect' and so on. Others refer to social characteristics: 'without documents', 'foreigner', 'IVF', 'medical', 'late child', 'paid childbirth' and so on. A newborn patient can have several labels at the same time, which are updated situationally depending on the organisational context, sometimes conflicting with each other or reinforcing each other's effects.

> About 2 p.m. we leave for N hospital, a call from the doctor-consultant, she says that she has just received a call from the chief medical officer and asked to go to the hospital in the neighbouring region, because there is a *severe* child on high-frequency ventilation since yesterday. It is a child weighing *600 g* with pneumothorax, on rigid parameters of ventilation. I hang up the phone and our chief medical officer immediately calls me back and tells me a story about this child. In the village a woman gave birth to a baby 600 g, a paramedic came to her (there was no doctor), he somehow contacted the administration of our hospital, because despite the fact that the woman gave birth in the neighbouring region, she has a *registration from St. Petersburg*. Although it does not matter (we have women from other regions giving birth and we do not transfer them). Initially they wanted to send our team there, but since everyone was busy with work and besides it is a different region, which is out of the city service subordination, nobody went there. As a result the baby was brought to one of the regional perinatal centres without intubation, breathing on his own. When

[doctors were] trying to warm him up in the ambulance, he received thermal damage to the skin (the child's skin is immature and rather low temperature plus compression of tissues easily cause burns). The regional transport service of the RAC could not take him out as they do not have a high-frequency ventilator.

We arrive at the perinatal centre, there are 3 doctors (2 local and one regional RAC) in the doctors' lounge. The doctor of the regional RAC (a woman about 30 years old, I may have seen her somewhere but I am not familiar with her) says that the child is very severe and *non-transportable*. I ask to show me the child. We go along the wide corridors, through the sanitary pass. The intensive care ward is large and spacious, but there are few children in it, except for ours, I think there is just one more. The doctor from this perinatal center says that she would like to transfer him, but it is impossible. I agree with her, but from a slightly different angle: 'we can transport him, but how much does he need it?' She replies to me that he has burns and they don't have a permanent surgeon, only a consultant who comes 2 times a week. We go back to the lounge, I look at the analyses and call the chief medical officer, saying that the child is extremely severe but I don't see the point of transferring him. She asks me more about his condition and asks 'if it was our [city] maternity hospital would you take him?' I reply that if he needs to be transferred, it can be done with our equipment. She says 'he would still have to be picked up (as he needs surgery and has a city residency). What did the surgeon write?' I read the report. After a pause she says to me 'go ahead and transfer him then!' This conversation is observed by doctors in the launge and nurses (the ones from RAC and regional). I say 'transfer'. Everyone in the room has doubts on their faces, the perinatal center doctor says, I don't think you can do it, but if you want to, go ahead and try. I'm off to get an incubator. There in the perinatal centre I meet a nurse (6th year medical student) who used to work in our hospital. He was happy that we are taking the baby: 'everything is fine here, but they don't know how to treat children in severe conditions – not at all!!!, maybe a couple of doctors and that's it. Will she [the doctor] leave tomorrow and what will happen to him?'. The baby's mum (*7 IVF attempts, frozen eggs*, first pregnancy) came to sign the papers. We transfer the baby to the city children's hospital, a baby tolerates the transport well (we manage to lower the ventilator parameters on the way). After 3 days he was stable with distinct positive dynamics (as much as possible for a baby of 24 weeks). (A participant observation diary, RAC unit, March 2020)

The significance of labels, as characteristics that determine treatment trajectories, is not the same. Some are part of professional communication and perform the function of additional coordination or particular attention. In the diary quoted above, mentioning that the baby's mother has undergone seven IVF protocols serves not only as a source of medical data but also as a marker of the social background of the patient and his family – that this is a long-awaited child and a long-suffering pregnancy. On the contrary, some other labels that seem to be social, such as 'old baby', also carry medical information, as they refer to a child who has been in the maternity hospital longer than usual, which may be due to the deterioration of an initially healthy child or a second wave of illness requiring transfer to a specialised hospital.

> Both Lena and Sasha are a bit surprised by some parameters reported by the doctor on the other side (a resuscitation baby, but '*old*', i.e. 5 or 6 days old) – Lena says that we will then go not to the initially planned maternity hospital, but to this baby, but on a new call. (A participant observation diary, RAC unit, July 2023)

Some other labels denote exclusively cultural data, reflecting common social stereotypes that are not related to medicine.

> And finally the last one [label] is 'karma' and 'alcoholics!' Why do alcoholics or drug-users have 10 children, while more educated people – 'have you noticed?' – have only one or none at all. – one or none at all (meaning unsuccessful attempts to get pregnant). At this point I was afraid that she [a RAC nurse] would ask how old I was and if I had children, but thank God she didn't (however, I would have fit into her theory). (A participant observation diary, ambulance RAC, June 2023)

One way or another, these labels reflect the emic system of categorising patients, which, among other things, is designed to facilitate decision-making on interaction with them for the medical staff. At the same time, there is a certain degree of polarisation of 'medical' and 'social' labels, depending on the severity of the child's condition; that is, the more severe the child's condition is, the less significant the 'social' labels become.

> At some point, a midwife came up to her [neonatologist of the maternity hospital] and apparently asked her to come to her department and examine the babies, as the mothers were waiting for her. The doctor Bella said that she couldn't come right now because she was transferring an *intensive care baby*, and that they had warned the day before that the weekend would be difficult (apparently not enough doctors in the hospital). And in general she didn't have time for '*paid babies*' (born in commercial department). The midwife said to her: 'what's the difference between 'paid' or 'free of charge' [childbirths]? Are there only two of you today (two doctors)?!' The doctor replied that there are three of them, but one doctor has to examine 50 children, and the second doctor does not get out of the labour room. The midwife stood in the corridor for a long time waiting for something. Then Bella quietly told me that commercial wards always ask to be observed first. (A participant observation diary, maternity hospital, October 2020)

The patient's ethnic 'label' is one of the statuses which, in addition to appealing to the opposition of 'friend or foe' and the exploitation of cultural stereotypes, is often associated with the bureaucratic aspects of providing medical care (for more details on this issue, see chapter 5).

> On the way to the call, we discuss that the number of maternity hospitals in the north [of the city] has decreased, and that the perinatal centre X. does not keep foreign children without documents (because no money comes for the health services provided to foreigners), but they cannot refuse to provide maternity care in childbirth – it is considered an emergency. (A participant observation diary, ambulance RAC, July 2023)

Although these dimensions are independent of each other and a 'child without documents' can have any ethnicity, at the stage of primary contact, these two labels are always compared, for example, the absence of documents is a reason for clarifying citizenship, just as a non-Slavic surname raises the question of 'documents' (primarily Mandatory Health Insurance policy).

> The nurse and doctor Lena continue to discuss non-Russians [patients]. They say all the time that the child (ours) is non-Russian, some kind of Easterner, although the mum is Russian and from Kursk region, it is obvious that the dad is *non-Russian* – they speak with some disregard. 'I don't like *non-Russians* and I don't like *boys*, I like *girls*', says a local nurse. I feel some indignation and ask finally how they determine that he is non-Russian. 'There, you can see it! He's hairy, look at his nose, his forehead. Russians can't be like that. You can see right away'.
>
> I look – well, he's really covered in fluff. Though I don't see any strong differences in anthropological features, so that they catch my eye. I look at patient's mum's surname and it's Armenian in origin. So they recognised the Caucasian nose and forehead. . . . I think: can a non-Russian child be pretty [for the personnel]? It would be good to look at a non-Russian but stable one, what they will say about him. . . . Then I think that these talks about common social fears are also a way to create co-operation in the conditions of hard and nervous work at the junction of two institutions. It's a local specific small-talk that makes specialists from different organisations, despite their discontent with each other, feel that in general they see reality in the same way. That's why everything is so supportive – apart from, apparently, the irritation about under-examined migrant women and their bureaucratic status. At one point a nurse complains to a local one that they have been slipped two '*illegals*'. (A participant observation diary, maternity hospital, July 2023)

However, in the absence of the need to maintain informal communication or during the process of the direct provision of care, the ethnic label may suddenly become irrelevant and insignificant:

> We stop by the intensive care unit of another children's hospital, Dr Sasha hands over the patient: documents, notes that the *patient is foreigner*, lists vital signs, '*Kyrgyz* passport with translation, then corrects himself – *Uzbek* passport with translation'. The local doctor replies 'I don't care'. (A participant observation diary, children's hospital, June 2023)

The ethnic label is expressed in such words as 'a foreigner', 'not ours' and '*kyzy-myzy*',[3] which often reflect narrow-minded ideas about the patient:

> In an informal conversation in the dining room, a RAC doctor, describing a severe case from her practice, calls a child '*kyzy-myzy*', thereby denoting his ethnicity. One of the nurses makes a remark to her, 'Well, you can't say that'! The doctor corrects herself, 'I'm in a good way, they are strong'. (Diary of participant observations, RAC unit, October 2020)

The ethnic label in this case reflects a fairly common notion among some healthcare workers that a 'foreign gene pool' is better, as they are not pampered by the benefits of civilisation. RAC doctors deal with children in need of emergency medical care, so the presence or absence of documents has practically no effect on the treatment and transportation process. On the other hand, the absence of migration documents and a mandatory health insurance policy for a mother from another country becomes a significant circumstance in other sectors, which is associated with the bureaucratic aspect and payments by territorial insurance funds. The doctors of a maternity hospital, which temporarily worked as an observational institution and accepted unexamined women without documents, described the unusual situation as follows:

> We are not accustomed to such a contingent. They are discharged on the second day, we ask staff to keep them longer so that at least the children can be vaccinated, but the obstetricians in no way agree. They say they must be discharged home no later than the second day [after delivery]. In the observational maternity hospital, mothers are discharged a couple of hours after giving birth. (Diary of participant observations, maternity hospital, August 2020)

If 'a child without documents' has no pathology immediately after birth, he or she receives a minimum amount of medical care and is discharged from a medical institution along with his or her mother. The situation changes when the child has signs of a severe disease or pathology. In this case, regardless of the presence or absence of documents, a child who needs inpatient treatment or long-term observation receives it free of charge, and the status (label) of the patient, given to the child by medical workers, allows the mother to accompany her child to a paediatric hospital.

Social labels such as 'IVF' (in vitro fertilisation), 'late baby' (born to a mother older than 35 years), 'medical baby' (whose relatives are medical professionals), or 'my friends' baby' often come up in conversations between medical professionals. They can have some influence on patient trajectories as well. For example, understanding the symbolic 'value' of a successful IVF attempt for a 'late-birth' mother, obstetric hospital doctors, in case of pathology, try to transfer the child to a large multidisciplinary hospital as early as possible. The 'value' of the child for the mother often emerges in the process of medical communication when, in addition to physiological indicators and the treatment performed, the IVF attempt number, the mother's age, or unsuccessful outcomes of previous pregnancies are indicated.

The combination of several labels for one patient may acquire the character of a conflict. An example below shows that the label of 'family births'[4] prevents the patient from moving into the category of 'resuscitation', as this has negative consequences for parents, that is, connection to a ventilator and separation from the child.

> It was planned to transfer a child to the neonatal pathology department from a large maternity hospital. The child was in the ward for '*family births*' together with relatives. When the RAC doctor came for him, he regarded the child's condition as extremely serious, requiring mechanical ventilation. As a result, a conflict arose between the doctor of the RAC and the doctors of the maternity hospital, who insisted that the child's condition did not require more aggressive therapy. As a result of lengthy negotiations, the child was transferred to a ventilator and taken to the intensive care unit in critical condition. (A participant observation diary, NRAC unit, October 2020)

In private maternity hospitals or in cases of paid childbirths doctors try to show parents that they are in control of the child's condition to the last minute, downplaying the significance of adverse factors and maintaining the overall picture of well-being, which is part of the service provided. An RAC doctor says, 'We were transferring a child with severe asphyxia and convulsions from a private maternity hospital, and the manager was saying to the parents at the same time, "Don't worry about so many wires on him. He'll be fine and go to school"'. Such behaviour, on the one hand, is aimed at reassuring the mother, but at the same time, it can create additional difficulties in communication with the doctors at the next stage, since the child is most likely to have an unfavourable neurological prognosis.

The presence of non-medical labels can be perceived by practitioners as a circumstance that complicates the work. In some cases, maternity hospitals tried to transfer children they could treat themselves under the pressure of parents – it was the reason. For example, in one of the maternity hospitals where children are usually transferred on the second or third day, the head of the department tried to transfer a child on the first day due to the fact that his parents (somehow connected with medicine) seemed to him '*troublesome*'; he said, '*they're kittle cattle*'. In another case, the label of '*a doctor's child*' or '*medical parents' child*' complicated communication between the doctor and parents:

> In one of the maternity hospitals, the parents refused to transfer the child to a hospital . . . all the relatives of the child were doctors. But on the second day, the child developed convulsions of unknown origin, and he was transferred to a [lung] ventilator, which made the parents agree to the transfer. The doctor on duty decided to speak with those parents, as she was told by shift that it was difficult to communicate with them. She said she noticed nothing unusual in the conversation with them, but they duplicated the information on the phone to the grandmother (children's cardiologist). In the pediatric hospital, the resuscitator on duty already knew that this was '*a doctor's child*' because the head doctor had called him and warned that the parents had contacted him, trying to organise the transfer on their own. (Diary of participant observations, maternity hospital, March 2020)

In this example, a planned transfer was delayed at the insistence of relatives with a medical background. They tried to influence the treatment trajectory using their knowledge and professional networks, initially refusing to be transferred to a hospital and be separated from the child and subsequently trying to influence the routing of the transfer. Communication between the doctors of the maternity hospital and the parents was complicated by the fact that, in the absence of productive dialogue, both parties acted inconsistently. In this case, the increased activity of the parents led to a delay in the transfer of 'a doctor's child', prolonging his stay in the 'unclear' status until the deterioration of his condition and the development of convulsions returned him to the original route of admission to a specialised hospital. Thus, an additional label caused a delay in routing.

For example, 'khlam' (bits and pieces) may refer to a child in a very serious condition who needs to be 'packed', that is, stabilised for a long period of time.

> On the way to the car and in the car (this time we sit with Sasha in the back) we discuss that the N. intensive care unit was 'punished' (they stopped transferring complicated patients there), as 'foetuses' died there more often. Sasha explains

> that it was not due to the work of the department, but because the most difficult children with negative prognoses were simply transferred there: there was '*khlam*' mostly, so unassembled! (Diary of participant observations, intensive care ambulance RAC, July 2023)

> In a conversation with the doctor Dima, who says that the child after vaccination 'collapsed – and we will not be able to assemble the child', we learn that to '*pack*' the child is not to prepare for transportation, but as the opposite of 'collapse', in terms of condition. (Diary of participant observations, children's hospital RAC, November 2023)

The word 'khlam' has a distinctly negative connotation and is therefore never used in the presence of patients' relatives or in official discourse. Within the community, however, it is more likely to reflect a state of disorder that requires a great deal of effort to 'order' and stabilise, rather than a personal characteristic of a patient. Most of the established labels in a particular sector are reflections of accepted practices and reflect the specificity of work specific to different stages of treatment.

> Doctor Sasha comes and says that it is necessary to go to the N. maternity hospital for '*noses*' (a child receiving respiratory therapy through a special device in the form of a mask or special nasal CPAP cannulas), but specifies that it is necessary to first coordinate this transfer with the head of the department, as she 'tears and swords' the nurse gets into the driver's seat, me with doctor Sasha get into the cabin, she insists that I should fasten my seatbelt and fastens it herself. (I note that in the other team, on the contrary, no one fastened it.) Sasha says, 'I don't like noses!', I ask her why? She replies that during the journey it is a less reliable system of oxygen supply and some malfunctions may occur. (Diary of participant observations, children's hospital RAK, June 2023)

Indeed, the doctor's fears are confirmed a few hours later during the transfer of this patient:

> 14.03 A nurse knocks at the window [between the cabin and a driver]: 'stop, please!' We are already not far from the hospital (I estimate 5 minutes away), but something must have happened. We stop, I can see that doctor Sasha and the nurse are doing some manipulations with tubes. (Diary of participant observations, intensive care ambulance RAC, June 2023)

CONCLUSION

The materials represented in this chapter make it possible to consider medicalisation as a flexible and mobile process, depending on the circumstances of a particular interaction, such as the complication of a patient's condition, organisational environments and the set of actors participating in the interaction, rather than as a linear and unambiguous mechanism for the implementation of medical power. As previous scholars of emergency care have demonstrated, medical triage or categorising patients might not be morally neutral processes (see Wamsiedel 2020; Dingwall and Murray 1983). Our materials show that medicalisation can be viewed as an optics, which medical professionals use to cut off information that interferes with making professional decisions in emergency situations (emotionality, lack of documents, connections, etc.), ignoring some of the information about the patient at that moment. In that way, medical labels like 'foetus', '500g' and 'defect', on the one hand, help to avoid the emotionally difficult details of the patient's condition, who is often on the verge of life and death, and on the other hand, they save time and effort of medical staff, reporting important information for the doctor and the medical team in the most concise way. In a situation of emergency resuscitation, this brevity is especially important since such labels indicate, first of all, specific medical decisions to save the patient's life.

The results of the analysis show that the non-linearity of medicalisation lies in the fact that the status of a patient, formed by professionals, is not limited to biomedical characteristics. The professional environment creates 'social' labels even for a newborn patient with extremely low agency, competing with an exclusively medicalised approach in this case. The registers of professionals' orientation to 'medical' and 'social' labels are switched depending on the severity of the patient's condition, which affects treatment trajectories taking into account the interests of the 'extended patient', that is, the 'child-parent' dyad. As medical professionals confront greater parental involvement in the interaction, they endow the infant with greater agency. For example, they understand the social circumstances of 'ageing' parents or parents who conceived a child with the help of IVF and show increased concern for the patient-infant, which in fact is a concern for the good of the parent. Labels like 'late baby' set a specific trajectory for the newborn based on sociocultural knowledge about parenthood. Thus, 'social' labels arise in the highly medicalised environment, even when professionals deal with a patient with limited agency. This mode of interaction partly competes with the biomedical approach, which dominates a deeply medicalised field such as inpatient and intensive care, and signals situations of 'demedicalising' relationships.

This chapter also illustrates the features of a moral career (Goffman 1961; Goffman 1963) in the case of such a specific patient, which is a newborn child with a diagnosed or suspected pathology. It does not include active conscious participation of the patient, relying solely on labels and categorisations produced by medical professionals. Parents, as part of the 'extended patient' (for a more detailed discussion of the concept see chapter 4), take only a limited part in shaping the child's trajectory. The following chapter will address this issue in more detail.

NOTES

1. 'Aspirant' is a term for a newborn with meconium aspiration syndrome, while at the same time it is a wordplay, as the word 'aspirant' in Russian stands for 'PhD student'.
2. In Russia, the middle name is derived from the father's first name and is used as a patronymic. Patronymics are more commonly used in formal conversations.
3. 'kyzy' is a part of a name for girls in some of the Turkic languages, while 'kyzy-myzy' is a pejorative wordplay pointing at a child's ethnicity.
4. A paid-for-service ensuring that a woman in labour can be with her partner during and after the labour

Chapter 4

Emotional Dimension of Neonatal Care

INTRODUCTION

There is a big celebration at the hospital. November 17 is celebrated as World Prematurity Day. On this day, parents and children who had gone through transportation from the maternity hospital, infant intensive care, and nursing in the hospital were invited to the hospital. Guests are gathering in the greenhouse hall. There, a festive performance awaits the children, but in the meantime, they can have a face painting applied. All characters are wearing white and purple. These are the official colours of care for premature babies. Parents are taking a lot of photographs, they are joyful and inspired and many are holding bouquets of flowers and gifts. Some bouquets are also white and purple.

The children appear to be between one and ten years old. It looks like an ordinary children's party – some are enthusiastically taking part in competitions, while others are crying and closing their ears with their hands. Families are gradually trickling in, and it is becoming crowded. Taking a closer look, you can see that many children have developmental disabilities, some of them are sitting in orthopaedic wheelchairs. Gradually, everyone moves into the large assembly hall, where the performance is to take place. Mushroom and Cheshire Cat decorations indicate that today they will be showing the children's play *Alice in Wonderland.* Soon the hall is packed out and guests have difficulty finding seats. Doctors and nurses are crowding at the entrance and the parents of their former patients are approaching them and giving flowers and sweets. The joy of recognition is shining on their faces.

A female official is speaking in happy tones on the stage. 'The joyful eyes of children are earned by doctors and parents, who have gone through and suffered a lot together', 'this is a holiday of faith, hope, love and victory over doubt', 'it's not only professionalism but also love and soul which were put into every child', 'high-tech equipment will never replace hearts, eyes and gentle hands', 'Napoleon, Churchill, Anna Pavlova were among the premature children, there are great poets and politicians, the future of our city among the children in this hall', she says. Her speech is permeated with appeals to the emotional and value side of medical care for premature babies. It is intended to evoke a feeling of pride in the doctors' work and symbolically actually emphasise its 'national importance'. She ends her speech by reading her own poem, in which doctors and parents are sacrificial heroes, who 'knitted their children's lives, unravelling their own ones'.

This heroic rhetoric is followed up by the next episode of the performance. A mini-film, edited by the intensive care unit doctors, is on the screen. It shows footage of the resuscitation transport service and the intensive care unit, accompanied by disturbing but inspiring music and photographs of surviving children 'then and now' with their birth weight indicated. This story culminates in a photograph of a baby born weighing 320g. The doctors are taking the stage to intense applause, many parents in the audience are standing up and have tears in their eyes. On stage, doctors are called superheroes.

The ceremonial part ends, and the performance begins. Many children are already tired, and families begin to gradually leave the assembly hall. They have an important task and are rushing to the departments. They are eager to see 'their' doctors and give them flowers and gifts. There is tea, sweets, cakes and perfume sets in the bags; one family has 'Wilberry' bags with blankets. One of the doctors is handing the cake and chocolates to a colleague of hers, saying, 'It is good for tea, and give those to the nurses.' In the corridor, a doctor is taking a photo with a child holding an inflatable daisy-shaped balloon. Another doctor is having a long talk with a mother, who is asking for his advice about vaccinations and nutrition. This holiday for the parents becomes an opportunity to renew contact with the doctors who cared for their children and whom they began to feel trust and gratitude towards.

Parents' gratitude is an important part of this recognition. On the walls, there are photographs of grown-up children who were patients of the hospital. Also, there are many grateful posts from parents in the hospital's social network group. The doctors who took part in focus groups admitted that personal messages from parents, who shared the stories of their children after discharge, were one of the most valuable and enjoyable aspects of their work.

The holiday is a ritual, which helps everyone feel part of a community. For doctors, this is a way to strengthen their own identity through public recognition of merit and glorification of their work. This is also a way of public channelling and display of emotions (for theory of ritual and its functions see Turner 1969; Durkheim 1995|1912; Marshall 2002). However, doctors and nurses often experience far more than just pleasant and publicly 'acceptable' emotions in their work routine. Every now and then, during fieldwork, they tell stories of doctors who 'took everything too personally' and eventually ended up becoming inveterate drunkards or committing suicide. One day, a random taxi driver, in a spontaneous conversation, told one of the authors of this book that he was a former 'burnt out' paediatrician. He had been working in an ambulance for eleven years before. Now he was working as a cabby but was thinking of taking some courses and becoming a massage therapist. The word 'burnout' came up in the field more than once without any prompting among interlocutors, too. Fatigue from work and its conditions, facing death and the inability to help and the need to talk about the serious condition of a child with parents are the invisible difficulties of medical work, which each interlocutor was forced to cope with individually.

Drawing on focus groups with doctors and nurses from different sectors of neonatal care and researchers' field observations of their work, this chapter examines the contexts of their emotional work that are usually implicit and hidden from the attention of patients, other health professionals, managers, officials and society as well as the state as a whole.

EMOTIONS AND EMOTIONAL WORK: WHAT ARE WE STUDYING?

Discussions about what we actually study when dealing with the field of emotions have been going on in the anthropological literature since the 1980s, and attempts have been made to define what 'emotions' actually are. On the one hand, anthropologists conducting research in non-Western societies have shown that emotions, the ways they are named and experienced, are largely determined by culture (Rosaldo 1980; Lutz 1986, 2011; Abu-Lughod 2016). This view was in contrast to the more universalist psychological and cognitive approach to emotion (Ekman 1980, 1984; Lakoff 1987; Levy 1982; for review also see Lutz, White 1986; Lindholm 2005). However, both anthropologists and cognitive researchers were concerned about the connection between emotions and language, that is, the so-called 'plane of expression' and the 'plane of content'. Emotions, to varying degrees, can be seen as cultural constructs, and they are often given to us in discursive expressions. Their manifestations are mediated by etiquette, rituals and various cultural conditions. Emotions can be understood in two ways – either as cultural categories or as embodied sensations (Leavitt 1996). However, the question arises: How do language and other ways of displaying emotions relate to experiences? How do they relate to the personal emotional experience being lived? Can a researcher access this experience (studying cultures that are distant and different from our own, in particular)? What does the anthropology of emotions study in this case (see review and discussion by Reddy 1997; Beatty 2014)?

This study deals with two types of data. Firstly, it is mostly discursive material entirely provoked by the research situation and obtained from focus groups specifically devoted to the topic of emotions. This conversation enables researchers to analyse the immediate terms and rhetorical structures which participants use to describe their emotional experiences. Secondly, the study includes materials from participant observation, which provides access to situations of spontaneous interaction where emotions are manifested, demonstrated, depicted and hidden. This occurs both at the discursive level and at the level of non-speech actions and non-verbal communication. This points out that not only communicative but also embodied emotions are present in the routine work of doctors and nurses (Lock and Scheper-Hughes 1987).

In both research contexts, both the research participants and the researchers conduct interpretive work: participants try to understand what the researchers want from them or how they should respond in a given institutional context and in a given work situation, while the researchers interpret their words and omissions, facial expressions, gestures, postures and so on. However, in both cases, people act within the framework of cultural conventions for expressing emotions and can also name and interpret them themselves. The researchers belong to the same culture and speak the same language, so they understand and recognise emotions and their symbolic and pragmatic meanings quite clearly. For example, talking about emotions turns out to be largely mediated by the cultural frame of the psychotherapeutic turn, common to researchers and participants (see Illouz 2008; Rose 1998). Observed emotions are accessible, among other things, through the intersubjective somatic mode of attention (in the terminology of Thomas Csordas, see Csordas 2002) and the empathic mechanism of cognition in anthropological fieldwork (see Fainzang 2007). Therefore, in contrast to cross-cultural studies of emotions, the issue of access to understanding emotional experience is not so acute in this study. At the same time, here we do not aim to discuss whether discursive or embodied emotions that are accessible to our observation and analysis are 'real' or 'true'. It is beyond the scope of this work to establish a connection between the 'plane of expression' and phenomenological experience as well as the authenticity of this experience.

Thus, this study tends to stick to the approach of the historian and anthropologist Monique Scheer, who, based on Pierre Bourdieu (Scheer 2012), tries in her work to remove the opposition between 'external' and 'internal' emotions and look at emotions more as a practice, because, like any other practice, an emotion is both spontaneous and conventional. The process of emotion production follows a practical logic, embedded in existing social relations, and relies on a learned, embedded habitus. Scheer identifies four types of emotional practices: mobilisation, or managing oneself and others through 'emotional contagion' and the cultivation of emotions (see Pirogovskaya 2024 on mobilisation of emotions among nineteenth-century physicians; on the political mobilisation of emotions also see Ahmed 2004); naming (interpretation and expression of emotions through discursive attribution, which makes them accessible to experience); communication (performance of emotions in interaction and reading the performance of another person); and regulation (working with emotions according to the rules of emotional display existing in the culture). A researcher can consider both the situation of focus groups and the direct routine work of medical professionals through the prism of this approach. For example, in a focus group, doctors or nurses may actively construct an image of parents as the main obstacle, egging on and 'infecting' each other. There they actively discuss and talk through the situations that cause the most acute emotional reactions, during which emotions receive form and interpretation. For example, during observation, a RAC doctor makes it clear to his team with his gaze and facial expression that the maternity hospital staff did something wrong, and his laconic performance is absolutely understandable for the RAC nurses (and for the observer as well). At the same time, in front of the maternity hospital doctors, the doctor restrains herself and, based on their corporate attitudes, does not express or show her irritation, although demonstrating irritation with the behaviour of a parent turns out to be quite acceptable.

Overall, emotional practices are considered in this work as an occasion to talk about the institutional tensions that arise in the work of doctors and nurses in different sectors, as well as to look at the structure of medical institutions and the construction of a newborn patient within these institutions through the prism of the emotional world of medical professionals. Contexts in which specific emotion management needs to be carried out also indicate the presence of institutional tensions because they must be contained and regulated according to certain rules. In a sense, doctors and nurses act like the flight attendants in Arlie Hochschild's classic work (Hochschild 1983), gradually adopting the 'professionalized' approach to emotions (Scheer's fourth type of emotional practice). Besides, for doctors, emotional work concerns not only communication with a client (patient/parent). Large resources are also spent on intra-professional interaction. Drawing on an interactionist approach to the analysis of face-to-face interaction (Goffman 1956), Hochschild considers how 'emotional labour' is carried out in a professional context, that is, how professional tasks influence emotional performance. This research shows that such management is carried out not only in relation to demonstrated emotions. It also concerns one's own lived emotions in accordance with the principle of medical detachment, which is closer to Hochschild's concept of 'emotional work'. Emotional work is done not only at the expressive and bodily level but also at the cognitive level, aimed at changing one's own feelings and attitude towards the situation (Hochschild 1979, 562). In a sense, the emotional work of medical detachment represents a specific professional 'technologies of the self', according to Michel Foucault (Foucault 1988).

Hochschild suggests that in modern society an individual tends to deal with his or her 'self' and emotions through interpretative frameworks that belong to organisations rather than to the level of individual experience (Hochschild 1983, 198). This study shows that the emotions of doctors and nurses (including difficult ones that require specific techniques) are provoked by professional activities in organisations, but their task of carrying out emotional work lies with the individual, since organisations do not provide special institutionalisedways of coping with emotions. One of the aims of this analysis is to survey medical detachment in a specific sociocultural context.

In what follows, it will be shown how the expression of emotions and work on them occurs in different institutionally determined situations and with different interaction partners, that is, children, parents and colleagues. Also, the differences between sectors of care and medical professionals of different groups will be shown. It must be borne in mind that access to representatives of different sectors was organised during the research process in different ways. For example, a focus group with doctors from specific hospital departments (e.g., RAC, intensive care unit, pathology department) was a single team, while maternity hospital doctors represented different institutions, which could affect the nature of their responses. There was no separate focus group with RAC nurses, although several people who participated in the focus group with nursing staff in maternity hospitals combined this work with work in RAC. At the same time, observation of the work of RAC doctors and nurses was available, as well as of doctors and nurses in maternity hospitals. The doctors and nurses in the intensive care unit were not observed in any way, and the nurses in the pathology department were completely excluded from this analysis, but there is a separate interview with the head of this department dedicated to the emotional aspects of her work. Such an arrangement of the material shows that it covers different sectors of care and different health professions quite unevenly, making it impossible to systematically compare them with each other, but the data are nevertheless sufficient to indicate and classify the various institutionally based tensions. The last part of the chapter will be devoted to moral assessments of the profession in the context of ideas about emotional burnout, mission and the boundaries of 'work' and 'personal' space.

PATIENT WITHOUT HISTORY

The third chapter brought up the issues of the joint work of medical and social labels and categories in the newborn child's development as a patient, and whether these categories have influence on the child's trajectory in neonatal care. Based on the results of the first stage of collecting and analysing materials, which resulted in the discussion presented in the previous chapter, we assumed that working with different categories of patients is assessed by medical professionals differently in terms of 'severity' and emotional involvement. Taking this hypothesis into account, the focus groups focused on how doctors and nurses in different sectors classified their patients and what the emotional aspects of working with each of these groups were.

Neonatologists at the maternity hospital are the first doctors who see and examine a child. They are the first to assess his or her condition and draw the line between 'norm' and 'pathology':

> It seems to me that there are children, who require your care, and you have to put in your effort and skill, and there are also those children, who simply need your assessment. You talk [to him or her], you put a stamp confirming he or she is wonderful, and [by doing so] you already pay some kind of, well, more empathy to the parents, yes, to the child. This is more than the use of your professional skills and abilities. (Maternity hospital neonatologist, female, focus group materials, August 2023)

Doctors draw boundaries between children they call 'understandable', on the one hand, and, on the other hand, children they call 'incomprehensible', or 'doubtful', that is, those who need to be observed in order to understand what interventions are required and what skills are to be applied. The group of children 'who need to be dealt with' becomes the point of application of exclusively narrow professional efforts. At the same time, the degree of full-term birth of a child, according to experts, does not directly correlate with his or her state of health. Although doctors single out children with extremely low body weight separately, the presence of clear protocols and action algorithms reduces the degree of uncertainty.[1] Even with 'severe' children, a professional knowledge of what kind of care needs to be provided to such a patient reduces the burden on the doctor. Tension is caused, first of all, by the need for medical triage and medical care in a situation of uncertainty, when nothing is clear about the patient, she or he does not have their own medical history and cannot describe their complaints themselves. It is the ability to identify deviations or 'abnormalities' in situations of uncertainty that seems to become a criterion for assessing one's own professionalism.

Doctors place children from consanguineous marriages, from 'ethnically' marked families and born to foreign citizens 'without residence registration' into a separate category. Such children not only may have a genetic pathology; apparently, they cause social anxiety as well, with them being aliens not only medically but also culturally, from the doctor's perspective.

Doctors begin to perceive 'understandable' children, as follows from the quote above, to a greater extent as subjects of interaction and consider them as part of the 'parent-child' dyad, in fact, giving the go-ahead (putting a 'stamp') for their socialisation as a normative citizen (see on the role of medicalisation in an individual's acquisition of 'biological citizenship' Rose and Novas 2005). It is worth mentioning that deaths in this sector of medical care are quite rare, and they are practically not discussed during focus groups with doctors and nurses of the maternity hospital.

Answering the question about emotions regarding children, nurses in maternity hospitals and RAC single out a separate group of 'unpromising' children. At the same time, they focus not only and not so much on the severity of their condition, but on the situation of their parents:

> Those, who have adequate mothers, are good ones. You hear stories that, I don't know, their first child died, then there were seven IVFs, then, well, a child is born, who is completely unpromising, and he is most likely to die as well, maybe, in a week or two or a month. Well, you listen to these stories, and feel uneasy, quite uncomfortable to work, because they want this child, they are fighting for him, but there is no chance. (A nurse of the maternity hospital and RAC, female, focus group materials, October 2023)

At the same time, both doctors and nurses separately single out a group of children of their friends:

> God forbid, of course, you be on shift, when it's a child of your friends, not to mention relatives. It sucks! This is even worse, well, I don't know about anyone, my head [at such moments] turns off, I can't think straight, I want to help somehow, of course, but if it requires your direct participation, and you have to do something with your own hands, well, it will be probably just a disaster. (A nurse at the maternity hospital and RAC, male, focus group materials, October 2023)

Empathy, as the interlocutors talk about it, turns out to be directed more towards the child's parents. A contact with the history of their family evokes sympathy, and direct acquaintance with them before the birth of the child sharpens the sense of responsibility. In both cases, it is the parents, not the children, who become the patients for health care workers, whose well-being they usually fight for. What interaction with a parent looks like and is assessed, as well as how such a 'distributed' or 'extended' patient is structured in different sectors of care, will be discussed in more detail in the next subsection.

It is necessary to add that 'difficult' and 'incomprehensible' children cause a noticeable feeling of tension among maternity hospital nurses. On the one hand, they apparently worry about their condition and well-being. On the other hand, such newborns create an additional burden on the maternity hospital staff, and if the maternity hospital doctor can completely delegate responsibility to the RAC transport team, the maternity hospital nurse cannot completely step aside and, in a sense, finds herself 'at the beck and call' of the RAC staff, helping them with diagnostic procedures and providing infrastructural support. Here's what a nurse said about a sick child who would not become stabilised:

> '[They] put on you [IVs and catheters], of course, you'll be sick for a long time', says the maternity hospital nurse to a child, who is being prepared for transportation by the team. 'Nothing good will happen', she adds, '[he's] not a fighter', she is disappointed. 'Well, where is your poop, you farted and that's it, you're not a serious guy'. 'Just pissing and pissing'. 'You've killed him and healed him [to death]', she says, apparently half-jokingly, addressing the RAC team. 'What a bully'. 'Poopy'. (Diary of participant observation, maternity hospital, July 2023)

The language used by the nurse in this fragment of field observation, as she is commenting on the patient's condition, is worthy of attention. She uses lowercase vocabulary and negatively coloured evaluative expressions ('a bully, 'not a serious guy', 'not a fighter') in relation to the child. She could use similar vocabulary in relation to any other child, but when she pronounces these lines, not only irony is heard in her voice and intonations but also disappointment and slight irritation that she experiences from this situation. The nurse emphasises the baby's 'doom' and the futility of manipulation and treatment. She has to constantly empty the container of urine and check for stool. It is an indicator of more normal functioning because the absence of stool indicates a more severe situation, which in turn means that the baby is not yet stabilised for transport. It is important to note that this conversation takes place during the summer vacation period, when the workload on medical staff increases. Moreover, it is going on after the team has been trying to stabilise the child for several hours, with the maternity hospital nurse on call. It is worth noting that some of the remarks are addressed not only to the newborn, who naturally does not understand them, but to the RAC crew, which indicates the impossibility of 'regulating' emotions (according to Scheer, ibid) and conducting emotional work in such a context.[2]

PIG IN A POKE

As was already described above, one of the results of the initial routing of a patient in the maternity hospital may be the call of a resuscitation team to stabilise the patient's condition and transport him or her to a paediatric hospital.[3] The peculiarities of the categorisation of children in levels of assistance are largely related to the specifics of this assistance and its temporary organisation. For example, in a maternity hospital, the peculiarity is that the doctor observes a 'patient with no history'. At the next stage, specialists receive a child with a short – but still some – history. This child must be stabilised and transported within a relatively short period of time.

'Transport' children (or 'planned', i.e., awaiting hospitalisation as planned) and 'regular intensive care'/'intensive' children do not cause anxiety and fear, since these are standard situations of care. However, 'severe' children stand out among intensive care ones. These are children with 'combined pathology', surgical pathology and developmental defects. They require more professional involvement and attention, since accurate diagnosis and neonatal care are not always possible in the conditions of a maternity hospital and its technological capabilities. In addition, a doctor, based on her or his experience, often predicts an unfavourable trajectory of the disease for these children. All children who 'don't fit into the scheme' also cause increased emotional involvement:

> I have an emotionally very difficult situation when, say, some not very clearly interpreted situation arises, when you begin to change something, add something, you don't get a clearly adequate reaction, and you understand that you are faced with the wrong thing. I mean you cannot rely on that, and this could be going on for hours. You are just telling me that some kind of pulmonary haemorrhage may begin there, there is a high dependence, there, on oxygen, that is a clear sign of some serious pulmonary pathology, while the pressure also decreases there, that is cardiac output drops, that kind of thing. When you can't find some kind of scheme that can push him in a positive direction, it [affects you] emotionally, for example, it's colossally completely [hard]. [. . .] Well, such a tense situation happens, yes. You have a feeling of your own [helplessness] like this, you can't take it in and get into the situation in any way. It's not right, it doesn't work out, it's not right again, it goes wrong, a clear picture doesn't add up in my head. (An RAC doctor, male, focus group materials, July 2023)

This fragment makes it clear that a doctor's emotional involvement is actually more connected with an increase in the degree of responsibility and worries for his own decisions and his own professionalism than directly with the patient as a certain individual entity or personality. A similar emphasis is typical in general for resuscitators in the intensive care consulting service and paediatric hospitals. The patient is seen rather as a more or less complex professional task – when the complexity is higher and more things go wrong, the tension rises and the more self-reflection is demanded.

Another category that is presented as complex in the discourse of doctors in intensive care is the so-called 'foetuses', that is, children with extremely low body weight:

> The foetuses for me still remain, well, excuse me for the word, it's 'lousy' [. . .]. In the previous hospital, we had no foetuses, we worked in a small hospital, and due to the bed shortage, we did not take children under a kilogramme. Therefore, when I came here, for me they were all the same. . . . I mean, I just looked at them fifty-three times from all sides, twirled them, look at something else if it's good or not, it's simple. (An RAC doctor, female, focus group materials, July 2023)

> Well, for me personally, working with children with extremely low body weight, who are 400, 500, 600 g, is also such a rather difficult threshold, because here you probably need a lot of practical experience, constant work with them in order to feel them. Because this is actually [. . .] these kids [. . .] this is a completely special thing. The maternity hospital staff is probably not ready to work with them either. (An RAC doctor, male, focus group materials, July 2023)

Prematurely born children with extremely low body weight not only have increased professional responsibility but also legal responsibility. In addition, they largely remain an 'unclear' category for doctors. For example, one of the interlocutors refers to the need to 'feel' them, to the ability to apply professional intuition based on extensive practical experience.

Another category of transported children, which is distinguished rather on logistical grounds and on the 'infrastructural' history of the patient, also contributes to the unclear state – it is an intensive care child who is transported by plane from another region. This, according to the focus group participants, is a 'pig in a poke', who can experience various fluctuations in condition at altitude, even if before that he or she was stable and ready to fly. Moreover, these children come from other regions where the level of neonatal care can differ significantly from the local one, so those children cause the sectoral specificity of 'emergency'. Besides, this example clearly shows that the degree of 'transparency' of the patient, just as in the maternity hospital, turns out to be the leading criterion of his 'complexity', including emotional involvement. Also, it is associated not with the lack of the patient's history, but with the possibilities of diagnosis and with the nature of the existing background of his history, treatment and routing.

During participant observation, it became obvious that another group of children, causing complex emotions, includes newborns with obvious genetic pathologies and a poor prognosis:

> The nurse says that the most difficult thing [for her] is to see children, about whom she says, 'Well, after all, it would be wrong to call them ugly freaks' (children with severe genetic pathology). She talks about a child with a big head, who had very thin arms, which even sensors for measuring pressure could not be attached to, and there was no way to dress him. 'The head and body are large, but the arms and legs are small, like a dwarf's'. As a result, they wrapped this 'poor child' in a swaddle so that he would not be cold. She says that such children fly home (meaning to Uzbekistan and Tajikistan) with their mothers to die. When she talks about difficult children, she almost cries, 'My heart bleeds. Such children cannot live. They'll suffer all their lives'. Also, she says that such children cause a waste of money, maybe someone else could be helped with it. However, she does not comment on any medical decisions or the mother's decisions in this regard. (Participant observation diary, ambulance, November 2023)

> The story that happened recently, and which, according to the doctor, caused a lot of emotions in her, is developing further. The doctor asks me how sensitive I am and shows me a photo of a child with a huge tumour on her head. Her mother was diagnosed with a pathology in utero, but she was told in a private clinic that everything would be ok, 'give birth!' The doctor condemns the clinic and the mother, regrets, and is indignant that this is a lot of money and resources being spent on a non-viable child. (Participant observation diary, ambulance, June 2023)

In both cases, medical workers are shocked by the appearance of the child, but for the nurse, the atypical body turns out to be more of a practical problem because it is impossible for her to dress the child, while for the doctor, it is a professional case, which she took a photo of and told her colleagues about. The nurse feels sorry for the child, who is doomed and will suffer, while the doctor, to a greater extent, complains about the decisions of the doctors and the mother, which led to the birth of the non-viable child. Both of them reflect on the costs and saving of resources (material, physical and moral) in connection with 'unpromising' situations. Apparently, this is a common rhetorical element for this professional community, emphasising their own values in connection with the principles of 'medical triage' of patients.

Unpromising children are those in whom not only financial ('governmental') resources but also professional and moral resources are invested:

> I mean you invest in a child, who, [as you] understand, obviously has no prospects; this is probably more difficult than investing in a child, who, as you understand, can still get better. You feel an unpleasant impression, though, even when you did everything well. (An RAC doctor, male, focus group materials, July 2023)

> We all worry about them, so that even such a difficult child, who still has no prospects in terms of [survival], and you still worry in the same way as you would for anyone else. Nobody wants a child to die in their arms. Accordingly, you work, you put in the same amount of effort to this child as to that child. (An RAC doctor, female, focus group materials, 23)

Doctors do not experience satisfaction from working with such patients. Moreover, working with them turns out to be very energy-intensive, because it turns out that to avoid deaths doctors have to put in as much effort as they would for other children with a more favourable prognosis.

It must be said that deaths in the transport sector of neonatal care with the current level of technology and equipment occur quite rarely. If doctors 'bury' a child (the term is used here to describe the dying process), then these are non-transportable children whose death occurs in the maternity hospital. One of the doctors notes that this is the most difficult part of the job for him:

> There are situations when nothing [. . .] works out, and it is clear that transporting the patient is completely ruled out for these reasons. I've had situations where you just emotionally can't leave, say, 'Well, that's it, guys, it's over here'. No, [cannot] put a stamp, sign the papers, and leave. Well, you just have to stay there practically until the end, at least to morally support the doctor, who continues to work with the child further, and understands that, in general, there is, in general, nothing more to do there, indeed. (An RAC doctor, male, focus group materials, July 2023)

On the one hand, if a child is recognised as untransportable, the maternity hospital takes responsibility for his death, and this death is included in its statistics. On the other hand, the RAC doctor in the transportation sector takes part of the moral and collegial responsibility upon himself in this situation, sharing its emotional severity (in some cases, according to the interlocutors, the doctor completely takes it upon himself).

It is necessary to note that, according to doctors and their terminology, children with pronounced genetic pathologies are contrasted with 'good' or 'beautiful' babies, who evoke a feeling of tenderness:

> Well, there are such cute kids, like little dolls that you want to take them, but sometimes they are not so nice. Well, this is, well, I don't know, it's so subjective, personal. I mean sometimes they are just so good, those with heart defects are always very beautiful, you see, for some reason. Just so good. [. . .] Those with asphyxia, they are usually just neat, okay, okay. They're simply so pretty. And they all are very [severely] ill, and very many of them have no prospects, because. . . . A big, fat, pretty one, he's so a little bit [sorry]. . . . The obstetricians made a fool of him. Or there is some serious defect that is known to be

> present in utero, and surgical intervention is unlikely to help him live better in future. (An RAC doctor, female, focus group materials, July 2023)

Often, 'beautiful' children only outwardly look not sick, but doctors understand that they have 'poor prospects', so such a dissonance of 'tenderness' and serious illness causes a feeling of regret. At the same time, doctors admit that they may be mistaken with dire predictions, and the situation may unexpectedly develop in a favourable direction:

> Oh, by the way, the foetuses [. . .] are very interesting children. There is probably a third-degree intracerebral haemorrhage. There is no need to harbour any illusions, when the brain tissue is torn there [. . .]. All the rest probably are okay, everything is very interesting [ambiguous] [. . .]. We saw in the hospital, when I worked in the hospital, sometimes they discharged neurological children, saying, 'You should just live with a neurologist'. Everyone said that, that kind of thing. And nothing happened. When he's one year old, he holds his mother's hand, comes with a cake, and says, 'I'm one year old'. You look and think, how come? . . . But apparently, such things, I mean it should have turned out to be cerebral palsy according to all other parameters, according to everything. (An RAC doctor, female, focus group materials, July 2023)

Such unfulfilled (for the better) expectations bring satisfaction, but doctors in the transport sector rarely encounter them since, as can be seen from this quote, if recovered patients and their parents return to see doctors, then this happens in the next sector of care. It turns out that in the transport sector, medical professionals interact with the child only for a short time, during which it is often impossible to understand his long-term prospects, let alone establish emotional contact with him:

> You may not even remember what the face looked like, you remember the excursion of the chest, and so on. Of course, you cannot become attached or take to the child. (An RAC doctor, female, focus group materials, July 2023)

Emergency physicians in the transport sector describe their professionalism by emphasising this brief and 'impersonal' interaction with the patient. According to this representation, if a child is considered primarily as a resuscitation case, only correctly made medical decisions and successful solutions of professional tasks can bring satisfaction from work and, hence, on the contrary, a task that could not be solved, according to the interlocutors, is taken hard as a professional failure.

BABY TALK(S)

During participant observation, special attention was paid to how medical professionals built communicative interaction with the child during the process of preparing for transportation. Speech statements addressed to the child, the so-called baby talk (speech register addressed to children, see Ferguson 1964), cannot be considered literally emotional work. However, this behaviour represents communication and performance of emotions (according to Scheer, ibid), which largely follows a culturally defined script. The categories of newborns that are relevant for a certain sector turn out to be related to the nature of communication with the child. Thus, doctors emphasise that if the child's health is satisfactory and he or she performs actions that are normative for that age (sucking, opening the eyes, moving), then the typical 'baby talk' begins. If the child requires active medical intervention, then 'baby talk' not only fades into the background, but it interferes with work. These words, in general, are confirmed by the data of the field observation:

> The transport team doctor comes into the room and examines the child. [He] immediately begins to call the child 'baby', [because he] turns out to be quite stable, pink (the doctor and nurse of the transport team are discussing his good colour) and even opens his eyes, 'he opened his eyes'. Therefore, he [the child] immediately receives many compliments like 'so good' and 'a fighter'. The doctor says, 'You are so beautiful. No matter you're a boy, boys should be beautiful, too'. When the child moves, while changing the IVs, they say tenderly [you are] 'being a bully'. (A diary of participant observation, maternity hospital, July 2023)

> The nurse transfers the child from the incubator and installs a catheter and infusion pump on the changing table, and wraps him. The baby cries, everyone begins to comment, 'Auntie is hurting you', 'Auntie has come to torment you'. (A diary of participant observation, maternity hospital, July 2023)

A transport child or a 'regular' resuscitation child evokes a desire to comment on his or her activities, as in this case, thanks to his movements, crying and open eyes. This occurs according to cultural patterns of interaction with infants and young children. Such a conversation is a sign to everyone that the situation is not difficult, it is routine, you can relax and joke, calm the situation. In the following passage, although the characters are the same – doctor and nurse as in the first quote above – the nature of the communication with the baby is sharply different:

> The child has low saturation and low blood pressure. The doctor of the transport team says that he is greyish and marbled. But when the lights are turned on, he appears to be more pink. In general, there are doubts about external signs. The

> transport team nurse looks into the diaper to see if there is stool and urine, but there is only one drop. The maternity hospital nurse is immediately asked to insert a urinary catheter. She says 'okay, it's a boy, I'll insert it. I would never do it to a girl, though'. (the participant observation diary, maternity hospital, June 2023)

Here, the volume of speech addressed to the child is falling compared to previous examples, and no one is 'babytalking' anymore. The child is interpreted as more 'severe' and 'incomprehensible' from a diagnostic point of view and requires more interventions. At the same time, he is under sedation and cannot express himself in the usual way a baby does. There are many IVs sticking out of him, which says that he is seriously ill. In this situation, the child is least 'humanised' and is not perceived as a communicative partner. He looks like a cyborg. His gender, in such a situation, turns out to be important not as a concentration of cultural stereotypes, as in the previous passage, but only in terms of medical manipulations.

Furthermore, sometimes in difficult cases, communication addressed to the child and, at the same time, apparently also to all other participants in the process, nevertheless appears:

> Transport service doctor, 'Stop fooling around, you're healthy!' 'The doctors at the hospital have been waiting for you'. 'You're [sitting] here with the girls, it's time to go to the boys! Don't you want to go see the boys? You need to come with us, the boys are waiting for you' (meaning that the transport team and the maternity hospital staff are women and the surgeons in the hospital are men). 'Well, baby, come on!'. (The participant observation diary, maternity hospital, July 2023)

After five hours of unsuccessful attempts to stabilise a difficult child for transport, during which there was minimal communication, the doctor begins to talk to him. On the one hand, this speech is a definite indication to surrounding colleagues about the nature of the situation. On the other hand, in some respects, this speech is reminiscent of addressing an inanimate object, such as, for example, a car that won't start or a computer program that won't work (compare 'come on!', 'what else do you want?'). This, in a sense, 'egocentric' (see Vigotsky 1939) speech has a certain self-organising function for the doctor in the difficult situation, when she is close to despair. In the end, when the child was successfully stabilised, the doctor admitted that she was nervous.

In addition to the categories of patients, the volume and nature of speech addressed to the child are also affected by the characteristics of the medical professionals themselves:

> The first nurse on the transport team interacts more with one of twin girls, who is more active. The second nurse interacts with the second girl, but she is calm and does everything almost silently. Therefore, I watch more the first one, who says during the manipulations, 'Girl!' 'Let's see, what you have here'. 'Let's be patient, little, poor thing'. 'Everything is good, my sweetie, it's over', she reacts to the crying and movements of the child, so that [the child] opens his eyes. They are discussing that the older one, although she weighs less, is more active. 'There's your bcgh, she's calm', their speech resembles classic baby talk. When the child takes off the mask protecting her eyes from light, the nurse says, adjusting it, 'Oh, you already give orders yourself!' The doctor of the transport team, a man, only touches the children, listens, and does nothing else. By the way, female maternity hospital doctors come up and also lisp with these girls, saying how pretty they are. (The diary of participant observation, maternity hospital, November 2023)

In this passage, one can discern gender differences in communication, determined by ideas about the cultural role of women. The male doctor does not use baby talk, although the babies he examines, are stable and active. In such a situation, more active communication with the child remains reserved for the nurse, who also fulfills the caring role assigned to her by culture and profession. By the way, the sex of the child turns out to be more important for nurses than for doctors. They note it and interact with the child based on this, while for the doctor, the gender is emphatically not important. Thus, two roles are constructed in interaction with the child, that is, the role of the doctor, as primarily a professional in his field, and the role of the nurse, as a woman caring for the baby according to culturally embedded norms.

'CHILDREN ARE CHILDREN'

The next sector of care, which the child is taken to is an intensive care unit. We have conducted focus groups with doctors and nurses at the hospital, where children with more complex conditions are usually hospitalised. The categorisation of children in this level of care is determined by slightly different specifics compared to previous sectors. On the one hand, there is an element of crisis and emergency, similar to the previous sector. On the other hand, the inpatient sector is characterised by a long stay for the patient.

Overall, children are called 'routine', 'standard', 'non-standard', 'critically severe', 'stable' and 'unstable', as well as full-term and premature. Doctors pay special attention to children who are difficult to diagnose and whose disease is severe and requires the doctor to make quick decisions that can determine the future prognosis ('urgent' patients). Unlike other sectors, 'old-timers' appear in the intensive care units of paediatric hospitals. These are children who lie sick for a long time, they can stabilise and then again become unstable and worsen. One of the doctors describes this situation the following way:

> When a doctor is faced with. . . . When staff is faced with such situations, of course, they don't not know how the matter will end, no one knows how and what will happen next, and this is a colossal emotional and psychological burden on a person, of course. On the contrary, there is another pole, though, when you see that everything begins to work out under the influence of your actions, your therapy, and the patient stabilises, [becomes] better, then wings grow, of course, yes. (An intensive care unit doctor, male, focus group materials, August 2023)

Some of the 'chronic' patients are gradually recovering, although, as doctors admit, their treatment is a labour-intensive and exhausting process. Others receive 'palliative' status, but doctors say that both groups (nurses call them 'adult children') are psychologically difficult for them to work with. It is necessary to point out that the category of 'unpromising' existed in other sectors, too, while the category of 'palliative' children appears here for the first time. Some of the children, after a long stay in the intensive care unit, are transferred to a children's hospice or orphanage.

> It is emotionally difficult for me to work with those children, who have no prospects. These kids are incredibly hard to work with. You know work doesn't disappear, and it turns out that it goes for us in circles, and you don't get any satisfaction. [. . .] I mean you leave in the morning and say, 'What have I done here?', even though I did a lot. And there is no gain. That's why it's harder with these children. (an intensive care unit nurse, female, focus group materials, November 2023)

> Well, you see, there is work, we still come to work, we have certain responsibilities, which. . . . We are not enthusiastic college girls, volunteers, who are touched by sick cats, dogs and others. There is work, palliative, and this is a certain part of the work that needs to be done well, that needs to be done anyway, that just needs to be done, and that's it. No matter if there is any meaning in it or there is no meaning in it, but if life and the state appointed us to do it, if we accepted these rules, if we chose this profession ourselves [. . .]. You just get mad from the fact that you are milling the wind, though. It's my personal opinion. (Intensive care unit doctor, male, focus group materials, August 2023)

Nurses and doctors in this sector describe their professionalism in a similar manner. They emphasise the futility of working with patients who are destined to die, but at the same time, they need to work and work flat out, 'to the end'. Meanwhile, doctors contrast themselves with enthusiastic ordinary people, who see value in such work, although they recognise that working with palliative patients is also part of the medical speciality. They criticise not the parents and medical colleagues who allowed obviously unpromising children to be born, but the current legislation, which determines the rules for nursing and resuscitation of newborns, and which they consider imperfect. Such patients cause regret and irritation because they take a lot of personal, emotional and professional resources from doctors, which is why there are fewer of these resources left for other, more promising patients, while, based on medical ethics, care is provided equally to everyone. Emotional work, human relations and communication are distributed evenly, at the expense of nurses:

> In my opinion, regarding palliative children, of course, a lot depends on our nurses, who are constantly [over occupied]. . . . You come and go, say, there are intervals, when no active actions are required, but the nurse is always busy. She is always with him [a child] and she continues [to look after]. . . . All the nurses, probably, whom I know, they still continue to treat them like children. They look after, they bathe, they talk [to them]. (An intensive care unit doctor, male, focus group materials, August 2023)

A specific problem of the sector, which creates a certain emotional background, is that the medical staff here, as they admit, do not see healthy children who do not need specialised help. 'I don't know whether they exist at all', says one of the focus group participants with a sigh. The most unconditional reward, or, as one of the interlocutors put it, a 'shock absorber' for doctors, according to them, is the recovery of children. On the one hand, doctors already emphasise the development of certain relationships with the child, speaking in terms of 'communication' with him. On the other hand, his or her recovery is seen primarily as an achievement of professional ambition, and 'not just emotions, that it's good for the child, it's good for the parents'. Nurses also point out that professional interest is above all – the variety of cases does not make the eye blurry. Apparently, treating oneself primarily as a purely high-level medical professional, engaged in extremely responsible work in the field of high-tech medicine, leads to the fact that there are practically no 'social' categories in relation to children in this sector. Everyone and everything is focused on a particular patient, who is viewed autonomously from his or her social environment:

> Children are children. And personally, I totally agree that children and parents are completely different, they are two parallels that [do not intersect]. . . . And love for children, mercy for children, compassion for children . . . have absolutely nothing to do with relationships with parents. Sometimes it's simply,

> most often, yes, looks like an ideal model, when this coincides with the relationship with children and parents. Sometimes, unfortunately, you are forced to keep some distance with their parents, but this does not affect your relationship with children in any way. Of course, you think about them during the day, at home, and at night. (An intensive care unit doctor, male, focus group materials, August 2023)

It is important that parents are still considered completely autonomous from the child in this sector of medical care. The visitation schedule is limited to two hours a day, and a child who is in intensive care status is largely alienated from the parent as an interaction partner due to sedation and devices. Although children lie here for a long time and doctors may develop a relationship of mutual understanding with them, the parent here (as in the previous sector) is not thought of as an expert on the child. Parent and child are perceived as separate 'therapeutic' units, which will be discussed further in the section devoted to emotional work in relation to parents.

BIRTH OF THE 'EXTENDED PATIENT'

The next stage of the neonatal patient's route is the neonatal pathology department, where children are either treated until discharge or, if there are repeated deteriorations, they can return to the intensive care unit (in some cases, they die there). Children from maternity hospitals can also be admitted directly to this department. This department is focused on a relatively long-term stay of a child who no longer requires urgent care but who needs to be provided with medical care and follow-up treatment, depending on his problems and pathologies.

The doctors of this department divide children according to the type of pathology ('genetics', 'asphyxia' and 'surgery'), according to the degree of full-term ('fat' or 'puffy' and 'seeds' or 'feeblings'), and 'relatively healthy', who seem the most 'incomprehensible'. The doctors endow these categories with subjective meaning, emotionally describing their preferences in working with this or that group:

> There are children, whom you empathise, you sympathise, if you can use such a word, and you try to help in any case, no matter how nice, loud, calm he or she is. Well, they are children, they cannot be blamed for their [illness]. (A doctor at the neonatal pathology department, female, focus group materials, September 2023)

Some people like 'flawed feeblings', others don't like 'screaming fat asphyxias'. These category names themselves seem to contain some kind of assessment, even if they are only part of medical humour. A special feature of this department is a more personal interpretation of children and medical labels because staff assigns children some character traits, noting their typical behaviour, depending on their pathologies or normal display. In a sense, children become not only patients but subjects of interaction, who do not exist here on their own. One of the interlocutors continues to develop the classification described above:

> We also have such a division as premature, surgical, cardiac, and neurosurgical children. . . . Well, we can go deeper. Also [they are divided into] large – small, heavier – lighter, with more complex parents and with less complex parents. Anyway, you have to work in tandem with a child and his or her mother. . . . Well, as you see both the mother and her child, some kind of interpretation immediately occurs. . . . This happens purely, apparently, on an emotional plane. You can approach someone several times, but for others once is enough. (A doctor of the neonatal pathology department, female, focus group materials, September 2023)

Almost from the very beginning of the discussion in the focus group, children in the classification system of department staff are associated with types of parents. In the quote below, for example, a doctor directly says that the work takes place with the 'parent-child' pair and this is somehow connected with the patient's assessment. The type and character of the parent seem to influence the state of the child. In fact, the parent and the child are united into one phenomenological unit:

> As a rule, children of normal parents are on the mend and recover faster. Some children of parents like these [inadequate], though, don't, because every day there's something new to treat. Their tests would show infection, or something. (A doctor of the neonatal pathology department, female, focus group materials, September 2023)

All subsequent statements by doctors in this department make it difficult to separate statements about the child from statements about the parents. They single out children of 'cool' parents, who are in positions of power (e.g., employees of certain government bodies and committees) and, traditionally, children of acquaintances and colleagues. However, even children who bear a primarily medical label are described through the prism of their interactions with their parents:

> Well, the most difficult thing is to work with children, who have a genetic pathology that you cannot influence at all. Very often this becomes an unpleasant news for parents, for example. . . . How to get this across to them, how to say it for the first time? Honestly speaking, for us . . . this is probably the most

> difficult thing both for parents and for us. I mean you are standing there and can't do anything. You can't remain silent and say nothing to them, you can't do that either. This is another unpleasant moment in our sphere. (a doctor of the neonatal pathology department, female, focus group materials, September 2023)

On the one hand, this is due to the fact that parents, as a rule, spend much more time in the pathology department. The hospital has a maternity ward, a day hospital and joint wards for mother and child. Even during COVID times, this order was not violated, and mothers were transported from the maternity hospital along with the child without being discharged home. On the other hand, the child here is more active, he is no longer constrained by resuscitation devices and medications. This not only gives the child the opportunity to express his or her temperament but also allows the mother to begin to gain parenting experience through caring for and interacting with him or her. Newborns without pathologies go through that in the maternity hospital, but here it happens for the first time, and a child with pathologies has the so-called second birth. Clearly, the formation of an 'extended' patient occurs, because here, finally, after transportation and resuscitation, the mother and other parents can be in greater contact with him or her, they learn to interpret his or her signals and understand his or her condition. We have not previously come across the term 'an extended patient' in the literature, but the first discussion of a socially distributed patient (such as a child-parent, a person with a psychiatric diagnosis – a member of his family, an elderly person – an accompanying person) is found in Talcott Parsons (Parsons 1951b, eg, p. 300). The same idea in research papers is discussed in terms of 'shared decision-making' in the case of the child-parent dyad (van Nistelrooij et al. 2017) or 'children-as-not perspective' (Clemente 2015, 16).

Another social category of children that is important for this department is 'maternity hospital children', whom doctors call 'pig in a poke'. On the one hand, children transferred from intensive care turn out to be more transparent and 'convenient', since there is enough information about them, treatment also has been selected for them, and they are transferred at the predicted time. On the other hand, it is equally important that parents of children who have undergone intensive care are much more prepared, and this makes it much easier for staff to interact with them.

Deaths of children do not usually occur in this department. Children are either sent to the intensive care unit or discharged home via hospice, acquiring palliative status. A more pressing problem is when a child is destined to become disabled. The severity of situations with a poor prognosis is also viewed by doctors through the prism of the need to talk with parents and convey to them the sad prospect. In the same way, according to the focus group participants, joy is shared with the parents, too. Here is a fragment of a dialogue, illustrating this moment:

> - We have longer, closer communication, also we experience their grief together with them, yes, and they warm to us, and we warm to them, we get used to the children, become attached, and then we have a very long communication, [because] for years we are together . . .
>
> - They send 'we are a year old' photos, there are nice words 'thank you, we are 6 months old here'. You look at the photo, and it gives you strength.
>
> - The reaction after discharge is quite pleasant, when you seem to have cured and sent away a healthy child, they have begun their own new life, and you have already faded into the background. Then suddenly, really, a year later, they send you a message, 'Don't you remember us? But we remember you! Here, hold it, we're sitting on the toy car'. It's incredibly pleasant, these are just a few people, but still they exist, such people. [Messages come] even from those people, those patients, whom you have already forgotten, and you think that they've definitely already forgotten you, suddenly they find your number, they're like that, 'How are you? We are calling you now, [no matter it is] two in the morning'. (Doctors of the neonatal pathology department, females, focus group materials, September 2023)

Moreover, this department is the first one, compared to other sectors, where doctors talk in terms of attachment to both the child and the parents. Although the successful outcome of work, which is embodied in recovered and normally developing children, becomes 'rewarding' in other sectors of care too, this is the place where long-term tracking of the child's further history takes place, and this happens through interaction with parents. The next subsection will be devoted to interaction and emotional work with parents.

WE EXPLAIN IN SIMPLE LANGUAGE

Parents, and mothers in particular, are not patients in any sectors of care described. Neonatologists, for example, describing their professional identity in contrast to obstetricians-gynaecologists, say, 'We absolutely don't care about the woman, but we are very concerned about the condition of her child'. Thereby they make it clear who is the object of their care. However, in all sectors, to varying degrees, doctors and nurses interact with, evaluate and discuss parents and, in some sectors, parents find themselves the central objects of emotional work rather than care. And certainly, in all sectors, the birth and formation of a child-patient occur with an eye on the mother and family.

Interaction with parents in the primary neonatal care sector is described as a very emotionally charged field, that is, almost like a battlefield, where doctors and nurses constantly expect threats, complaints, defiant behaviour and excessive demands for attention from parents, so they describe parents' complaints as inadequate to reality:

> I'm putting a [drip into] a vein for the child, and she [the mother] is standing outside the door. Naturally, the baby's crying loudly. I'm telling him something like that, 'I understand you're in pain'. . . . But I'm talking to the child calmly. I don't know, it seems to me that everyone does the same [. . .]. Then suddenly she starts screaming wildly, flies in, grabs my hand, then runs to the head of the unit, shouting something weird, sort of she's telling my child he's in pain, and they're going on injecting him anyway. This is where the commotion and fuss begin [. . .]. So, they wrote a complaint against the head of the unit and several other doctors. (A maternity hospital nurse, female, focus group materials, October 2023)

Nurses emphasise that they try to avoid conflicts with parents and do not tell them any medical information, which they are not sure of, as they don't want to expose themselves to harm. Both doctors and nurses say in unison that in the view of parents they are 'pests' and 'Gestapo', although they try to explain this by the emotional state of the woman and her family after childbirth, because if something goes wrong with the child and he or she is not be discharged home and everything will not happen according to the expected scenario, the parents may not be able to immediately accept this and blame for this situation those, who do not give permission for discharge.

The patient's extended family is presented as a major problem and burden because extended family members and grandparents, asking for details over the phone, take up valuable time and distract from work. The fathers are described here anecdotally. For example, one demanded to be present during resuscitation, but fainted, later he threatened a doctor with a pistol but burst into tears. Here is how, for example, the situation that happened in the early 1990s of the last century, during the heyday of crime, is described:

> I come in the morning, he [a newborn's father] says, 'Explain to me in simple language, just in simple language [what's going on].' Well, I did. Then he is taking out a wad of money and a revolver, 'Choose! What do you want?' It's what he said to me, 'What do you want to get? Get either a bullet in the forehead, or take the money and do something'. Can you imagine? Well, after I actually explained it to him in a simple language [straightforwardly], he fell down with this money, with the revolvers, and began to cry. (A maternity hospital neonatologist, female, focus group materials, August 2023)

Working in a tense emotional context is portrayed as part of the image of a profession, which requires overcoming not only misunderstandings of relatives but also real dangers, both legal and quite 'physical', in order to devote time to a patient. The ironic use of the phrase 'explain in simple language' illustrates the difficulties of finding contact with parents, who are almost in an altered state of consciousness.

Speaking about the misunderstanding and difficulty of contact with parents, the interlocutors note that some mothers claim to be experts in medicine ('I read it on the Internet'); they try to control the actions of the medical staff, walk around with a voice recorder and require individual attention, especially if there was a birth paid. However, they are completely unprepared for the birth of a child and do not understand how to feed him or her and what to do if he or she sleeps. But parents who refuse treatment cause the most irritation:

> I can also add something about interaction with parents. . . . Erm. . . . I caught myself thinking at some point that I got very angry, when a woman turned down treatment. I just, I don't know. . . . I feel an avalanche of anger washing over me. At the same time, of course, [I understand] I'm talking to a normal woman, and I'm sure I know how to do it properly, I know what's best. But you [mother] are doing harm now, and I've got an impression I'm appropriating this child for myself thereby, because I'm making the decision for his mother, I know what needs to be treated, but she turns down this treatment. It's hard for me to talk to a woman, who takes down, for example, treatment. (a maternity hospital neonatologist, female, focus group materials, August 2023)

If a mother refuses treatment, she thereby shows distrust of the doctor and questions his actions, but first of all, according to the neonatologist, she threatens the child, that is, the one who is the neonatologist's patient. By doing so, she deprives the doctor of the opportunity to demonstrate his or her professional competence. When a child born in this sector requires neonatological care, there is a trade-off between the mother's right to be included in the parent-child dyad and act as an extended patient making decisions for the child, and the child's right to be an individual patient of the neonatologist, and, accordingly, the right of the neonatologist to make independent medical decisions. This quote confronts the doctor with the need to reflect on the mother's subjectivity and her own right to 'appropriate' the child in such situations.

Despite such interactions, saturated with conflicting assessments and emotions, as it is described, doctors also talk about the need to seek contact with the mother, build relationships with her, and explain to her the situation.

During participant observation, researchers could indeed observe episodes of communication between neonatologists and mothers:

> A mother is coming to the intensive care ward to see her child, who is not being transferred. She is very young and seems completely calm. She is standing and looking at him, trying to touch his cap and blanket. Then she is coming out, and as she sees the head of the intensive care unit in the corridor, they start talking. I can only hear a few words, but the mother is asking questions for a long time, and the head of the unit is explaining and commenting patiently, in detail, on the child's condition in medical terms (however, it is not known how clear they are to the mother). Their dialogue continues for about twenty minutes, although the head of the unit looks very tired. (the participant observation diary, maternity hospital, June 2023)

Such interaction shows that the doctor considers the conversation with the mother as her duty and, despite fatigue, does not refuse her communication and explanations. At the same time, doctors complain that they do not have the education, developed skills and proper training for such communication:

> It seems to me that, in fact, we have an insufficient level of psychological education or the ability [opportunity] to devote as much time to this [issue] as a psychologist, a competent person, because anyway, I think our communication and successful communication with a parent is personal experience. I mean we talked many, many times, we came to a common opinion on how to act effectively, and, therefore, we went on communicating according to this effective model. Until every doctor [. . .] finds these keys, he can't hit it off with the parents, [nothing will come off]. I mean this is a second specialisation, which no one has a diploma in. (A maternity hospital neonatologist, female, focus group materials, August 2023)

It is necessary to note that the doctor, contrasting herself with the psychologist and emphasising the lack of a psychological diploma among medical workers, actually includes the performance of a psychological function in understanding her own role in relation to the parent. Thus, she includes this in the performance of her own identity. At the same time, maintaining such an image, doctors switch from complaining about parents, who take away their time and resources with their importunity and incompetence, to regrets about insufficient contact with parents:

> It happens that you do such a huge job, but you see child's parents [very little time]. . . . You only come to them to sign papers – one, two, three, just such a pile of all sorts of consents, papers for all sorts of drugs. Then they [patients] are [taken to and] treated in the hospital for a long time, and there they see the

> effective work of the doctors, but it looks like nothing happened here, as if it was something trifling and petty, rubbish. [The parent can say] I felt bad, my child felt bad, and we were separated, that's it. (A maternity hospital neonatologist, female, focus group materials, August 2023)

The lack of subsequent feedback and gratitude from parents, although justified, nevertheless does not allow the doctors to feel recognition of their own role and the result of their own work.

During the focus group, nurses also switched from criticising parents to talking about their own role in teaching the mother basic skills to handle the baby. Here is a fragment of one dialogue:

> - I love them very much, I treat them sort of . . . [I tell them] listen, here you wash your hands, then you'll change clothes. They [mothers] are like this [timid], sometimes they are . . . they are very afraid of premature babies, and if you begin to show, they follow. . . . You need to push them there and say, 'Do you know how important it is that you're talking to him? He hears you. You want him to get better, don't you?' And then you begin this 'blah-blah-blah', and then gradually, she also begins to do something. . . . It's very [difficult to talk to] fathers . . .
>
> - Three hours later you go out into the corridor, she is still there.
>
> - Let her stand there, I don't mind!
>
> - I like this, I like teaching women, but we don't do that very well either. . . . I can, well, I mean I like to talk to them. In principle, I can, if she is adequate, say, yes, I can [communicate] . . .
>
> - We have these open boxes. You sit and see everything. If anyone walked by there, I can clearly see. You showed her once [what to do], and that's it. It's your child, you wash his butt and love him. I'm sure even the most empathic infant nurses could not do better than his mom, more tenderly and correctly. No one can do [care for] a child better than his mother. (Two maternity hospital nurses and a nurse from the maternity hospital and intensive care unit, focus group materials, August 2023)

Nurses thereby emphasise the role of the mother in caring for the child, which is placed at the forefront. The second remark, however, belongs to a male nurse, while others are made by women; nurses engage in a certain dispute with him, highlighting the importance of the female gender role, which they see as part of their own professionalism. They also emphasise their desire to socialise a woman into her new status as a mother, to carry out emotional work with mothers, communicate with them and reassure them ('he hears you, do you want him to get better?') However, as a rule, only 'adequate' mothers deserve that kind of trust. Health professionals in all sectors of care also use this basic categorisation of 'adequate' – 'inadequate' in relation to parents.

It must be borne in mind that what is said during focus groups may not fully reflect the actual practices of medical staff. Rather, these materials demonstrate how the interlocutors understand and enact their own professional identities, what aspects of work concern them, and what meaning these images and issues take on in collective discussion. It is not known for certain what the practices of interaction between neonatal doctors and nurses in the maternity hospital and parents actually look like. The researchers could only see the arrival of the transport team. But it can be assumed that those practices differ from their discursively created description, just as in any other fragment of social reality, what a person says does not always coincide with what they actually do. For example, the following small fragment of observation in a maternity hospital clearly shows that nurses perform not only a socialising function in relation to the mother but also act as an authority who provides or limits the mother's access to the child:

> A mother of another child from the intensive care unit looks into the room twice, but he does not yet require transport. The maternity hospital nurse tells her twice that they won't let her in until the 'severe' child is transferred. The mother comes up and is worried the transfer of her child. We spent several hours in the maternity hospital, but she was not allowed to see the child, although the room was spacious, and she would not have physically interfered with the work of the team. (The diary of participant observation, maternity hospital, July 2023)

The nurse does not have 'objective', that is, institutionally determined reasons for not allowing a mother to see her child (violation of the visiting regime, quarantine or other medical reasons), but she acts as a person institutionally vested with power. By not allowing the mother to approach her child, the nurse makes her life easier because it is a way for her not to create unnecessary disturbances, not to waste unnecessary resources, not to carry out emotional work, as well as to demonstrate concern for her colleagues on the team. Such actions by the nurse are situational and, apparently, depend on institutional conditions, namely the lack of staff in the maternity hospital at that particular moment. The nurses of the transport team also display similar situational power over the mother:

> A mom in a leopard-print robe is coming in, with eyelash extensions and with the latest model of iPhone in her hands, and she is asking me with gestures, quite carefree (no one else's paying attention to her), whether her child is in the incubator. I'm nodding. Then she's asking with gestures again if she may take photographs. Just then the brigade nurse reacts and says that 'photography is prohibited'. The mom is not very upset and is leaving the room at once. I ask

> the nurse why she didn't allow it. She replies that this is really prohibited in this department (it turns out that there are even notices about the ban on photography and videography), but in her personal opinion this is not necessary, 'Well, why does she need this? Why does she take pictures of "such" [a poor child]? To cry in the evening?' (The participant observation diary, maternity hospital, July 2023)

The nurse in this excerpt demonstrates control over the mother's actions, citing official prohibitions, but at the same time rationalising her actions through reference to concern for the mother's feelings. Perhaps, in addition, the nurse reads the mother's habitus as class-alien or too frivolous, inappropriate for the role of the mother, and thereby tries to 'put her in her place' within the framework of the possibilities available to her.

'MUM, DON'T CRY!'

In the above-mentioned sector of resuscitation mobile teams, medical workers have minimal interactions with parents. The responsibility to communicate medical information about the child rests with the maternity hospital doctors, and only in the most severe cases do the maternity hospital doctors ask the team doctors to take on the task of explaining what is happening to the child. Employees of the resuscitation and advisory service say that they usually only briefly explain to the mother which hospital and which specialists the child is being taken to. Here is an observation fragment illustrating the distribution of communication with a parent during the preparation of a child for transportation:

> A mom comes, she is a fragile, beautiful woman of about 35, holding her back and stomach, walking with a limp, as if overcoming pain. She reaches the ward and, on the threshold, begins to cry and turns away. The maternity hospital doctor and the transport team look at each other, saying, 'Well, everything is clear' (apparently, assessing the mother's condition as 'inadequate'). But she soon returns, having pulled herself together. She is looking at the child from afar, from a distance of a couple of meters, and crying. Neither the doctor and nurse of the transport service, nor the head of the intensive care unit of the maternity hospital tell her anything. This silent scene is taking place in complete silence. But suddenly the team nurse breaks the silence and begins to talk to the mom! She says that her child will be taken to the hospital and gives the number. The mom asks if they are doctors, who will treat her baby. The nurse replies they aren't. 'We are a transport team, we only transfer. Our service is invisible, but don't worry, we take care of all the children as if they were our own. We remember everyone. Don't cry, he's doing well'. The mom says she understands her and she is crying with joy! Seeing that the mother is more stable than she seemed to be at first, both the transport team doctor and the maternity hospital

> doctor join in the conversation. The head of the unit, who had previously displayed her temper, complaining to colleagues about work problems, answers the mother's questions in a completely calm tone – the child receives food, formulae for children of his age, 'the neurosonogramme says everything is within the age norm'. (The diary of participant observation, maternity hospital, July 2023)

This fragment shows that the appearance of the mother in the ward causes all doctors to intensively work on interpreting her moral state; that is, they are trying to assess how 'adequate' she is. In such a tense situation, the nurse of the transport team takes on the task of defusing the situation and showing a 'human' attitude towards the mother, thereby carrying out emotional work, which the doctors are trying to distance themselves from. She reassures and consoles the mother, explaining to her the simplest things about transporting the child, and such communication allows her to place the mother's tears in a different frame. The woman is not in hysterics, she is quite consciously crying with joy. This frame switching (see Goffman 1974) allows doctors to safely interact with the mother and tell her about her son's health, because she is recognised as 'adequate' and communication with her, thanks to the intervention of the nurse, will no longer threaten the doctor. The neonatologist at the maternity hospital, in turn, takes control of her own temperament and talks to the mother like a professional. At the same time, for the nurse, who initially takes on the communicative work, performing this task is also a way to construct or increase her own status both in the eyes of doctors and in the eyes of parents.

Here is another example illustrating the role of a nurse in a child transport situation:

> A mother is coming into the room. She looks quite calm. The transport team nurse is asking if she held the baby in her arms. The mother answers 'no'. She is given her child, already swaddled for transportation. She is holding a bundle with her child and begins to cry. The nurses begin to exhort, 'Mum, just don't cry, take care of the milk!'. They ask what her children's names are. We are getting ready to go, we are going out into the corridor. The doctor of the transport team, who previously filled in the documents, comes back and asks why we are not leaving. 'The mom's holding us up there'. She [the doctor] says 'you could've done without it'. Then, upon returning, she said disapprovingly, but without explanation, 'Mom there . . . was like that [inadequate]'. (the participant observation diary, maternity hospital, RAC department, November 2023)

In this fragment, nurses not only do emotional work according to corporate norms ('no tears') but also demonstrate that they play an important role in the socialisation of the mother. They let the mother hold the baby for the first time, encouraging her to take care of the milk. In fact, they go against the will of the doctor, who for some reason regarded the mother as 'inadequate', and protect the possibility for her to contact the child. Probably, the doctor's logic is provide specific care for the mother by limiting her contact with the child; that is, she does not see the child in poor condition and does not have time to become attached to him if something bad happens to him later.

Team nurses can contrast themselves with maternity hospital doctors in a similar way:

> They're wrapping up the children, then they bring in their mother, she's in a wheelchair and her leg is bandaged. She's holding the girls in her arms – one, then the other, for a long time. She is quite calm, sometimes she tries to cry, but rather out of joy. The more active girl apparently had not eaten for a long time. The mother asks if the children will be fed before leaving. The maternity hospital doctors, young women, say that they don't feed them on the road. But the nurse of the transport team, a woman of retirement age, takes the bottle with milk and begins to feed the girl, who is hungry. She says that she feels sorry for her [child]. Then the doctor invites the mother to feed the second one, but the little one does not suck because she is not hungry. (the diary of participant observation, maternity hospital, November 2023)

The nurse, who begins to feed the baby contrary to the arguments of the doctors, demonstrates her great cultural competence. She is much older than the young employees of the maternity hospital, and this is a certain symbolic resource that she emphasises with her actions. As an older woman, who already has not only her own children but also grandchildren, she knows better what the child needs. She confirms this with both actions and words ('feel sorry') and shows an almost motherly concern for him, in contrast to the more formal approach of the young female doctors.

Sometimes doctors also take on emotional labour. Apparently, this depends on the composition of the team (including gender, because men, as the examples showed above, are less prone to emotional communication) and the individual characteristics and temperament of its employees:

> Meanwhile, the child's mother's coming into the room. The team is going to transport the child soon. She is standing next to him, pale and lethargic, then begins to cry. 'Mum! If you cry in the room, we'll kick you out!' says the transport service doctor. 'There are only positive emotions here! Do not cry! Don't spoil the aura! You mustn't cry, you must save the milk!' Then the doctor softens and tells the mother that children feel emotions, so she shouldn't cry. The mom asks where they are taking him, the doctor gives the number of the hospital with cardiology. 'Everything will be fine, everything will be fine', she exhorts the mother, but does not say anything about the child's condition, and, trying to distract her, asks, 'What did you name the child?'. Later, in the

> elevator, she admits that she hates to see moms crying because 'it's annoying'. (The participant observation diary, maternity hospital, June 2023)

This fragment clearly shows that the ban on tears is fully implemented. On the one hand, a mother, who cries with joy after childbirth, or a mother, who cries, worrying about the condition of her child, are culturally normative scenarios for the manifestation of emotions. However, in this institutional context, they turn out to be unacceptable since the doctor has to spend resources on emotional involvement, while her tasks include, first of all, professional assistance to the child. Therefore, the mother's tears are seen here as a threat to the moral well-being of the doctor and, consequently, to the physical well-being of the child and generally as a violation of the social order. Crying should be stopped immediately by using various techniques, such as threats, distractions, exhortations or ceremonial reassurances such as 'everything will be fine'. At the same time, if it is customary to hide irritation from the actions of colleagues in another sector, then it is acceptable to demonstrate it to some extent in relation to parents. Showing irritation with parents' behaviour becomes part of professional and corporate communication, just like, for example, discussing patients.

In the discourse of doctors at the intensive care consulting centre, parents are usually described as people who can be blamed for the condition of the child, their patient. These are mothers who are not examined or do not decide in favour of an abortion in the presence of obvious pathologies. However, there is a ban on making such accusations:

> There are mothers, who did not go anywhere [attend antenatal clinic], did not treat any of their illnesses. Alright, then what did they want? Of course, we never say it out loud, we only say it to ourselves. (A resuscitation and consultation department doctor, female, focus group materials, July 2023)

Doctors assume that the mother is responsible for what happened and feel angry and upset about this, so they carry out some emotional work on themselves and restrain their emotions in accordance with corporate values. Meanwhile, during the focus group, doctors seem to be trying to reconsider their accusatory rhetoric and come to the defence of the mother and her decisions. One of the doctors says:

> Personally, in such moments, I let it go, on the one hand. The first thought that arises in my head is, 'What have you [mother] done? Who needs that?' On the other hand, this is her choice, this is her story. (An RAC doctor, female, focus group materials, July 2023)

Like the maternity hospital staff, during a focus group, transport doctors eventually come to the need to discursively justify the behaviour of mothers, even though some irritate them or actualise the definition of 'inadequate' during their direct interaction:

> We don't know because they are all different, yes. Someone comes just like that, saying, 'Where should I sign?' and doesn't even look at the child. 'Where are the papers?' She puts a squiggle and that's it. And she doesn't even [cry]. . . . 'Yes, that's it, is he already being taken away? I see, I'll go then'. And that's it, nothing more. There are such stories. Things happen. This doesn't say anything about this [mother]. . . . Of course, you can think something [bad] about this mother. For example, 'Well, in general, she's kind of a bigot'. But in fact, no one knows what will happen with her in a day, because her hormonal levels are changing. Now something bad has happened to her family or some other things, so [she is like that] . . . (An RAC doctor, female, focus group materials, July 2023)

An attempt to explain the mother's condition occurs both by referring to the emotional background, which is under the influence of the past birth (we met this explanation in the previous section), and through an attempt to suggest 'social' reasons for her indifference or any other inappropriate behaviour. In these fragments, a kind of discursive work with emotions (irritation, indignation) and discursive reconciliation with mothers takes place, while outside of this situation, those emotions are considered rather an obstacle to the work of the RAC transport team.

EVERYTHING WILL BE FINE, RIGHT?

At the intensive care unit, communication between medical staff and parents becomes more regular and systematic. Here, it is no longer possible to do without detailed explanations and building long-term relationships because the child can stay in intensive care for a long time. In addition, the child's prognosis in this sector is already becoming more or less clear, so in some cases, this requires the doctor to carry out specific communicative and emotional work to convey bad news. In this sector, at least at the level of focus group representation, doctors become more responsive and understanding towards parents:

> If we talk about this, there is such a big problem, because all women go to the maternity hospital for a healthy newborn. Therefore, when something happens, it is such a difficult situation that . . . I mean [she has] bought diapers, baby vests, she [doesn't expect something bad] . . . she is surrounded by all sorts of

> bows, booties, hats, etc., but her child was taken to the intensive care unit in the first hours of life, and on the fifth day he was not discharged home. And, of course, this is, in fact, a colossal stress for the family. You often have to share it with child's parents, especially in the first days. (An intensive care unit doctor, male, focus group materials, August 2023)

> The problem here is, of course, in parental infantilism. We have a lot of people here [among parents], who are psychologically completely immature, who are faced with such a challenge that, in general, you wouldn't wish on anyone, which rarely anyone can endure in her life, really [. . .]. Of course, they behave [inadequately], well, and probably have the right to behave in a wide variety of ways. Alas, a doctor in this case, of course, is just such kind of a buffer. (An intensive care unit doctor, male, focus group materials, August 2023)

In the first fragment, the doctor talks in terms of sharing emotions and a stressful state with the parents. He constructs himself as an empathic person, who realises both the mother's expectations before the birth of the child and her shock from the collapse of the normative scenario. In the second quote, on the one hand, the doctor begins to accuse the parents of infantilism, but then immediately justifies and emphasises the gravity of the situation, which they find themselves in. If the medical staff of the maternity hospital finds the infantilism of parents a certain practical problem that can be solved by socialising the woman who has just delivered a child into the role of a mother, then in intensive care, parental immaturity, together with the ordeal that befell them, is interpreted, rather, in existential terms.

In the intensive care sector, as in the case of doctors from maternity hospitals, the interlocutors talk about those fantastic ideas and perceptions that parents glean from the media or the Internet, but here doctors are ready to take responsibility for those problems and misunderstandings, false claims, interpretations and hopes that arise in communication. The same interlocutor continues:

> Avicenna said [. . .], 'Look, I have two opponents – you and your illness. Now you are against me, and I am alone against your disease. If you are on my side, then we will have two, and it [the disease] will be alone, and we will definitely cope with it'. When a person understands that in fact he is not talking to the enemy and you are on the same side of the barricade, no matter what happens. . . . Sometimes this changes the situation a little. But, on the other hand, you know, [. . .] often we, the medical staff, ourselves create the biggest communication problems [. . .]. Because when a person hears contradictory information from doctors, [. . .] for example, they hear one thing from obstetricians, they hear something else from neonatologists in the maternity hospital, but here they are told something else, you know. Or it happens that here one doctor told them one story, and another doctor told them another. The doctors

may have told the same thing, just in different words, but the person psychologically clings to all sorts of inconsistencies, [so] distrust is born in his head with all the ensuing consequences. (An intensive care unit doctor, male, focus group materials, August 2023)

The doctor talks about the responsibility of all doctors, whether primary care or intensive care, for the integrity of the picture that develops in the parent's head, and the need for dialogue with her or him. Maternity hospital doctors talk in a similar way about finding the key to communication with parents. Therefore, everything depends on successful communication with the parent because it can lead, at a maximum, to successful treatment and, at a minimum, to relief for everyone during the difficult period of the child's stay in intensive care. At the same time, parents may not only misunderstand or misinterpret the words of doctors but also directly blame them for what has happened to the child:

'How did you treat him? You killed him with antibiotics. Or, [you] ruptured his lungs with ventilation!' They say, 'How can you explain to me [to the parent] that rotten lung tissue, it [. . .] from any ventilation, can rupture, right?' Well, these are the moments [that irritate], and you have to use your vocabulary explaining it to them this way and that. I mean I use examples, tell them about everything we [do]. We inflate balloons, try to come up with any clear ideas, in order to get it across to [parents]. (An intensive care unit doctor, female, focus group materials, August 2023)

Doctors build their image around their own moral integrity and steadfastness. Even in the case of such accusations, which they perceive as unfair, doctors remain true to their principles and try by all means to achieve at least some degree of understanding from the parents.

This kind of communication and emotional labour comes at a cost:

In fact, every child and the family of that child, who ends up in intensive care, they have the right to receive sympathy, empathy, compassion. This is a normal feeling that should [. . .] be received by a member of this family, for example, parents, grandparents. [. . .] They each come with hope and with a request that we will provide them with this sympathy, empathy. Here, in fact, a very big problem arises, because our main task is to cure their child. And very large physical and moral resources are spent on this, because there are things that we sometimes cannot voice, but we understand all the risks, we do not voice them, or any of our fears [. . .]. Certainly, the doctor cannot emotionally withstand, for example, the entire amount of communication with relatives of their patients, [. . .] after all, you need to communicate with each patient based on his level of intellectual development, moral, and psychotype [. . .]. There are parents, who really need pathophysiology, and there are parents, who don't need it at all, absolutely. [. . .] And the problem is precisely in the fact that there are no resources to answer them in simple language. (An intensive care unit doctor, female, focus group materials, August 2023)

By sympathising, empathising and, most importantly, trying to speak the same language with the parent, the doctor wastes his or her valuable moral resources, which should be intended for the child. The doctor does not say this directly, as it was said in the maternity hospital sector, and frames it much more carefully and caringly, but nevertheless, the multiplicity of requests from patients' relatives turns into a problem that doctors can no longer cope with. A separate difficulty is the need to switch between different 'psychotypes' of relatives, their different conditions, from depressive to aggressive, and, accordingly, between emotional modes. At the same time, the doctor saves his or her emotional resource by not reporting all the facts and prognoses, and hiding part of the disease picture from relatives.

This is how the picture of interaction with parents is described in terms of responsibility, which has a complex configuration:

This is also a common story, even for all mothers and fathers, it happens often . . . after they have thrown out [negative emotions] what they think needs to be thrown out on the medical staff, they naturally begin to punish themselves, pick at themselves, and so on. Therefore, it is very important to say, 'Look, it's not your fault directly, but whatever we all are doing now is [for a good cause], we try to just get out of this vicious circle, and we often walk in the dark, not taking in what'll happen next, but we keep going. And more often we bring it off'. (An intensive care unit doctor, male, focus group materials, August 2023)

Doctors say they are trying to relieve parents of guilt, in fact acting as psychologists, although they suggest that, albeit unwittingly, some responsibility may lie with the mother, who was not attentive enough to the child's health. Also, doctors take on a significant part of the responsibility – this is responsibility for delivering bad news, for the condition of the child, and for his or her death:

It's one thing when he'd been dying for a week, his parents had realised that and they were just waiting for your call. That's one situation. Completely another situation is when they [newborns] somehow suddenly die. Of course, this is much harder, because you have to explain it, because it seems to the mother that she saw [her child] yesterday and everything was fine, although nothing was good from a medical point of view. It seems to her, though, he was alive, moving his arms and legs, and then you call her at eight in the morning and say, 'He, unfortunately, died, his heart couldn't stand it'. [. . .] First, they cry loudly into the phone, then they begin to call you back. Again, it is much easier if she

> didn't see him before that and her child arrived from the maternity hospital already in critical condition and died within a few hours. Well, of course, she knew that they were taking him away, that he was bad [severe], but she didn't see him and such things did not happen. . . . But if he was lying for some time [by her side], she also was taking part to this process of treatment, emotionally, and then he unexpectedly died within a day, this is [terrible]. Also, sometimes it happens that a month after death they [parents] can text you something. You begin [to make excuses]. . . . You shouldn't do this, I know, but it still somehow slips through, well, as if you're making excuses. To tell the truth, you have nothing to justify yourself for, though. You thought you gave the child a chance, but this chance may not have existed. (An intensive care unit doctor, female, focus group materials, August 2023)

Reporting the death of a child is one of the most difficult responsibilities assigned to an intensive care physician, because it is the department where most deaths of children occur. It is difficult to call such an action routine, since it requires a lot of work with emotions, and takes up a lot of time, as can be seen from this quote. Also, the doctor latently feels the need to justify herself and make excuses to the child's parents for this death, trying to relieve herself, at least rhetorically, of responsibility. In fact, she should not have felt this responsibility because the death of the child did not depend on her efforts and was a foregone conclusion. Emotional work in this case consists not only in regulating her own emotions in relation to parents, in confronting their experiences, but also in the fact that the doctor has to resolve moral dilemmas within herself and at the same time be in a complex dichotomy between feelings and obligations. Thus, the most difficult professional responsibility for the doctor is not to give parents false hope:

> Because, in the end [it can be worse] . . . it seems to me when I come across parents, it happens very, very often. . . . I mean you can fall into a conversation, talk [about] an absolutely difficult child, talk about the pathology, about further outcomes, but in the end you will be questioned, 'Well, everything is fine, right?' All [parents] just try to get you to say everything is fine. And you are forced to explain that the child is in the intensive care unit. [This means that] no, not 'everything is fine'. 'Everything is fine', when the baby was born and now is lying on the mother's breast. But sometimes they directly demand this [confirmation] from you. (An intensive care unit doctor, male, focus group materials, August 2023)

According to social studies of medicine and medical communication, some doctors believe that it is better for the patient to hold out hope that the diagnosis is not final. Thus, doctors give way to their own tacit hope that their patient does not have a terminal disease. 'The regime of hope' for patients (in our case, relatives) means doubting the reliability of the facts known about the disease and searching for alternative or new methods of treating it and making large-scale investments in this. Staying in the regime of hope gives them some more period of more or less 'normal' life outside of palliative status. 'Regime of truth', according to this concept, means that a person recognises the incurability of the disease and trusts existing proven methods of palliative support. Other doctors, according to the study, adhere to the idea that the regime of hope is unacceptable and leads only to negative consequences, but nevertheless they are faced with the fact that patients have their own perspective, which cannot simply be ignored by imposing a regime of truth on them. In our case, doctors also face the need to balance between two regimes. Although they clearly prefer the regime of truth, in practice, in complicated communication with the parents, it turns out to be difficult for them to implement it (for the discussion of the regimes of truth and hope in communication between doctors and patients see Ferrie and Wiseman 2019; Salander, Bergenheim and Henriksson 1996; Moreira and Palladino 2005; Petersen, Seear and Munsie 2014; Robinson and Hunter 1998).

The focus group with intensive care unit nurses was quite short. It took place in the morning, after the end of their working day. The shift turned out to be difficult, many children were admitted to the department in a difficult condition, the nurses were tired, and the conversation was very short. The participants did not have the strength to go into details. In a sense, such a field failure is largely illustrative – it shows that nurses in the intensive care unit are under a colossal burden of caring for children, which is repeatedly emphasised by the doctors themselves, and their exhausted state after the shift only confirms this.

It is nurses who bear most of the responsibility for accompanying the child. They cannot leave, unlike doctors, and therefore, by their own admission, they try to avoid interaction with parents in order to somehow save their own energy. At the same time, nurses prefer to communicate with those parents whose children have been in intensive care for a long time because they are already used to it and behave 'calmer'. Parents of newly admitted children are 'psychologically unprepared' for the birth of a sick child and tend to 'vent' their emotions on nurses. Therefore, out of corporate solidarity, nurses warn each other about which parents to watch out for:

> In the morning we hand over our shift and say, 'Here are wonderful parents, adequate, nice, everyone understands. Nobody comes up to this child. And the parents of this one are weird. Be careful there, there are inadequate people there, they don't perceive requests, they don't perceive anything else'. (An intensive care unit nurse, female, focus group materials, November 2023)

Nurses say that the best time of their work was during the COVID quarantine, when parents were not allowed into the department. If intensive care doctors consider talking with relatives part of their job, then for nurses the child is their only patient and object of care, and parents only interfere with their work. The difference in the interpretation of giving and gratitude from parents is also not surprising. For example, one nurse says that upon discharge, 'they try to forget us, like a bad dream, parents really try to forget this'. On the other hand, doctors note that parents send photographs of their recovered children, and this serves as an important moral reward. A doctor jokes that 'these photo reports do not allow me to go to work for Yandex Delivery'.[4].

'PARENTS ARE A SORE SUBJECT'

'Ninety per cent of our work is parents and paperwork,' employees of the Department of Pathology of Premature Babies characterise their work this way. As already mentioned, communication with parents is most intense precisely in this level of help. 'Back to the topic again, right? Parents. It's a sensitive, sore subject. No one complained about the children, only about the parents,' said one of the doctors, when the attempt to return the conversation to the categories of children failed.

There is a branched classification of parents here, which is no longer limited to a simple division into 'adequate' and 'inadequate'. Doctors distinguish, for example, a group of parents with a difficult social status, that is, drinkers, a group of those who can abandon a child, a group of graduates of orphanages. Sometimes department employees intervene in the family's social situation and ask the guardianship authorities to check it. Another group is the parents of children who were transported to the department directly from the maternity hospital, bypassing intensive care. Such parents are unprepared, make more claims, are not ready to accept the situation of hospitalisation, and often refuse it:

> [Those, who come] from maternity hospitals, they really don't understand the seriousness of the situation. This begs the question, why did they just go to the hospital in the first place? RAC staff have spent time visiting maternity hospital. We also have spent our time, reagents, and nerves here. (A doctor of the neonatal pathology department, female, focus group materials, September 2023)

Such parents waste the material and human resources of two sectors of neonatal care at once. The biggest problem, however, comes from parents with a certain 'boorish' habit:

> Now [there is] some kind of layer that is very demanding, taught by the Internet, a neighbour, a girlfriend. They know how to demand from doctors, what to demand, what they have the right to. They believe that they can open the door with their foot and talk to you like a service person, who owes you everything, and you should only smile in response. (A doctor of the neonatal pathology department, female, focus group materials, September 2023)

> I like people with some good manners, I don't mean mannerism. But it seems to me that people should communicate in a certain way. And this is [intolerable], when they open the door with the foot, this is the wrong behaviour, you know, when they shake you, when they grab doctors by the chest, you know, and they supposedly show you up in your true colours. This is some kind of rudeness, this, you know. One of them is standing there, chewing gum, covered in tattoos, you know. 'Well, so what?' he says to me. I answer, 'Nothing, let's take a seat'. You see, [. . .] well, that is sort of cattle. (A head of the department of neonatal pathology, female, focus group materials, September 2023)

Doctors complain that such patients' relatives view medicine as a service, and the doctor must do emotional work like that done by Arlie Hochschild's flight attendants (Hochschild ibid) and any other service employees. According to their categorisation of parents and assessment of their behaviour, they largely echo the head of the department (see the second quote). There is a separate interview with her, where she actively contrasts polite and ill-mannered parents. Thus, such a division, as well as the requirement of respect for oneself as a professional of a special kind, can be considered part of the corporate culture of the department. The 'boorish' behaviour of parents requires specialists to have specific skills in regulating their own and others' emotions in interaction. Some of the interaction stories, as in the maternity hospital sector, are told in the following genre:

> So, we coped [with the child's illness] somehow, and two days later she [the mother] says, 'Can my husband come today?' I say, 'Of course'. I didn't think that he wore a holster. Well, then she comes [. . .] and says, 'You know, this is not my girl'. Imagine, she told me that, when her husband came, 'This is not my girl. When I was in a coma, I saw a completely different child'. Then her husband takes out his pistol and grabs me like that. The head [nurse] was not taken aback, she called for help, and the guys from the intensive care unit came running. [. . .] A colleague from the intensive care unit told me then, 'The contingent is such that it's time for the heads to give us service weapons'. Well, later this father, however, came there with a bouquet and said, 'You're normal!'. I say, 'Thank you very much!' He sounded like, here you go, you've earned it, [here's] a bottle of vodka and a bouquet of flowers. (A head of the department of neonatal pathology, female, focus group materials, September 2023)

Such stories, on the one hand, create a certain image of a profession, wherein one has to work almost under the threat of physical harm emanating from a specific 'contingent'. On the other hand, as in the maternity hospital sector, these success stories are told about conflicts with parents, when the doctor, as a rule, triumphs and proves that he or she is right, when he or she is able to neutralise the threat and emotionally 'steer through' the situation.

Monitoring the personal time that the doctor devotes to communicating with parents constitutes a significant part of the discussions during the focus group. So, the central question is whether parents should have the doctor's personal phone number, and each doctor makes his or her own decision – some give it only to 'adequate' parents, others get a separate phone number for them. Over time, some people completely abandon this method of maintaining contact.

Recently, measures to support doctors have been introduced institutionally. To conserve medical staff resources, parent question time was officially limited to one hour per day. But unlike the intensive care unit, the presence of parents here is perceived by doctors rather as a positive factor:

> When they are here, when they see what is happening to the child, when it happens before their eyes, say, some kind of deterioration or they see some kind of manipulation, then they perceive it differently, easier than when they don't see, or judge by words. Supposing, I'm forced to call and say, 'Today we have a worse situation there, and so on, so forth'. Parents still perceive it differently than when they see the child, when they are here, present during some deterioration. (A doctor of the neonatal pathology department, female, focus group materials, September 2023)

> [A girl] has grown, [. . .] two kilogrammes, she has already put on some weight there, she was supposed to be discharged, literally the day before discharge, her mother says, 'I'll come and lie down, be by her side, I'll be lying down with her just for two nights, and then [we both] go home'. Okay, then she comes and lies down, and that night the child's intestines twist, and she is taken to the operating room in a generally pre-terminal state. They barely pulled her out there, fortunately our resuscitators are excellent. So that mother and I later became friends, [. . .] and she says, 'You wouldn't believe me, if I hadn't been there that night and personally been present and seen that she ate at six in the morning, and at seven she turned grey and her stomach puffed up, I would have thought that you had done something. I would never in my life have believed this could happen out of the blue'. (A doctor of the neonatal pathology department, female, focus group materials, September 2023)

It turns out that the presence of a parent in the ward is not necessarily a hindrance and a waste of time and resources for medical staff. If a parent sees what is happening to the child, observes his or her conditions and the manipulations carried out by the medical staff, then trust in the actions of doctors and the doctors themselves increases. This also facilitates communication between the doctor and the parent because no additional explanation is required in this case. COVID times, when visits were limited and it was necessary to maintain contact by telephone instead of personal meetings, are now assessed rather as difficult times, when the emotional burden on doctors has increased compared to the normal situation:

> You can't imagine what was happening here during the COVID era. In general, at that time, we didn't let parents in, they didn't let mothers in. And we made a decision for ourselves that we would give [mothers] our personal numbers and send video greetings like this to each mother every morning. We filmed the kids, I mean there are twelve to fourteen children there, you have to go on a round in the morning and record from twelve to fourteen video greetings, send them to their mothers, answer a bunch of questions, which they have, of course. 'What is that a tube in the mouth?' [. . .] 'You took a picture today, but the light somehow fell wrong, and he's not pretty today, but he's wearing a sock from yesterday'. (A doctor of the neonatal pathology department, female, focus group materials, September 2023)

Doctors actually had to spend more time on communication, responding to the complaints and concerns of parents, who could not assess the situation using video recordings and be constantly in touch. However, ultimately, the doctors in the focus group came to a positive assessment of this experience:

> - You know, from time to time we are asked to look at the child. [. . .] I come to see the child, mom, dad, grandmother, grandfather are sitting there. And they all sit there and say, 'You know, we . . '. I can't even speak . . . [holds back tears]. 'We lived', she says, 'from one of your videos to another. And then we re-watched it a hundred times'. And they pronounced this in such a way that they just brought me to tears, this is it, and you think that. . . . Well, you don't even think that you [spent] some ten minutes there. God!
>
> - Do you remember them creating groups for us! So, this is your group, 'you are Maria Ivanovna, great, you were included in the group'. You look at the group and there are dad, mom, grandma, cat, dog, and you. . . . My gosh, it was, of course, [unbelievable]. . .
>
> - And everyone sends emoticons, emoticons, emoticons, flowers, smiles, hearts! (doctors of the neonatal pathology department, female, focus group materials, September 2023)

Doctors complete this reasoning in terms of reciprocity – most relatives are grateful people who value the resources of doctors and their participation. For a small contribution to supporting parents, the doctor receives a reward both in the form of emotional recognition and in the form of subsequent photographs of growing children, as already mentioned. In fact, doctor find themselves included in the baby's extended family, at least for the duration of hospitalisation, and sometimes for a longer period because warm relationships with mothers that have developed in the department sometimes turn into friendships.

(NOT) PLAYING IN TEAM

In addition to difficult and recovering children and adequate and inadequate parents, the work of medical specialists also includes interactions with colleagues. These contacts also require emotional work. It is very important to mention that the nature of those relationships ultimately determines not only the moral well-being of the doctor and the team as a whole but also, in some cases, the material and professional resources available to the newborn patient. The interactions of health professionals with each other can be divided into communication within the same work team and between representatives of different sectors of care.

Doctors in the transport sector describe the mobile ambulance team as a single organism, a team that must work harmoniously while travelling to another institution:

> Yes, we have a doctor and a nurse, and it's not like in the department. We have a doctor, a nurse, and a driver. They are a single whole. Nothing is ideal, of course, it depends on the driver, though [good/bad driver]. . . . Well, it's sort of a little different, our team is something completely different. And this interaction is very addictive. It differs a bit, this is not a hospital, and for everyone who has ever come to the car, if you stay there, it is very difficult to leave. [. . .] We have a slightly limited car space, yes, completely different relationships with each other. And human relationships are completely different, because the space is very small. There is a doctor and a nurse in the department. They have completely different divisions of labour and different relationships. Our relationships are more, say, in my opinion, closer, because we communicate more closely, specifically with the person in this car. (an RAC doctor, female, focus group materials, July 2023)

The relationship between team members is described by the doctor as close and reliable, having its own specifics compared to a regular department and less hierarchical. There is an informal hierarchy of doctors and nurses in the department. Some are considered more competent, while the work of others causes criticism from colleagues. This problem is solved by assigning doctors and nurses to calls for patients of varying severity. Those who occupy a higher place in the informal hierarchy usually go to a more complex child.

Doctors at the intensive care unit describe relationships within one team as teamwork, too. If any contradictions arise, they are only about the treatment of children, and they are resolved collectively:

> - We have some issues among ourselves, when some contradictions [arise] in terms of treating children, for example. Someone sees the situation like this, someone sees it differently, a third person comes up and sees it the third way, i.e. yes, sometimes you have to come to some common denominator together, consulting with almost the entire team.
>
> - In fact, there are no irreconcilable contradictions in the team. And the strength, say, is with the doctor. . . . The strength of the doctor lies precisely in the fact that he can admit that he doesn't know everything, call on other colleagues for help, and everyone together can help to solve this problem, attack it and cope with it later. After all, our department is a team game, because alone, of course, you can hardly cope with the tasks that life puts before you. (An intensive care unit doctors, male, focus group materials, August 2023)

Doctors prefer to replace the term 'conflict' with the word 'misunderstanding' and resolve these misunderstandings in a working manner, thereby describing interaction with each other as extra-personal, exclusively professional. By the way, the same is true for patients in this sector. Here, doctors emphasise the special value of nurses as part of a professional team:

> Well, in general, all the work, in fact, in my deep conviction, 90% of success in intensive care depends on the work of the nurse. Well, the doctor is like this [secondary]. . . . The main job, of course, lies with the nurses. Those children, of course, [are exhausting] and the lion's share of the efforts to care for them, to bring them into 'marketable form' and condition, is done by the nurses, because every now and then you can leave this post and do other things, and the nurse, who works with this child, cannot. (An intensive care unit doctor, male, focus group materials, August 2023)

The doctor emphasises a respectful attitude towards those lower in the hierarchy, thereby creating an image of a team that values each of its employees, regardless of status, since each employee is a high-class professional.

Nurses in the same department also prefer to describe the relationships and difficulties of interaction in a team in terms of 'work moments'. Even if someone [of colleagues] is 'annoying', it turns out that everyone is 'trainable', that is, the contradictions are resolved over time:

> Sooner or later we all get along well, becoming friends, right? Well, we're not close friends, but we do the same thing. Of course, there are conflicts. Even not conflicts, but misunderstandings. Well, our work is hard and it can be difficult to control emotions, sometimes conflicts arise, yes, nobody's perfect. Well, some squabbles happen. (An intensive care unit nurses, focus group materials, November 2023)

Nurses here also prefer the term 'misunderstanding', but admit that their interactions with each other can be emotionally charged and that it can even lead to verbal altercations, even though they prefer not to share their own emotions in this regard and the details of how these relationships are regulated. They do not mention whether they have any complaints about the doctors or the department's hierarchical system.

The doctors of the pathology department, who also form a single team, speak about their own colleagues in a similar way:

> A diverse female team is a difficult collective and it's always sort of a compromise. It is clear that very often there are clashes and misunderstandings. (A doctor of the neonatal pathology department, female, focus group materials, September 2023)

Such responses hint at the fact that emotionally tense relationships may arise in any team but, on the other hand, there is a degree of sincerity that employees of the same team afford each other and the researchers. They behave in an emphatically correct and respectful manner towards colleagues and acknowledge that problems arise, both with each other and with their superiors, but they refuse to discuss conflicts publicly.

In both of the latter cases, they talk about internal relationships with a smile, which makes it clear that the participants will not 'wash dirty linen in public'. All of them understand what situations they are talking about, but they protect the face of each other and the team as a whole. As far as the head of the department is concerned, she can already afford to speak out more directly. 'The head nurse can be terribly annoying, because the heads are special', or 'I don't expect to be liked by everyone, I can be quite tough, sometimes there are very difficult conversations', she says. Her narrative contains colourful stories about conflicts with subordinates, about the betrayal of colleagues ('stab in the back') and about her own educational work with the team that she carries out. Different ways of talking about relationships in a team in the case of intensive care may be associated with the difference in the prevailing emotional styles (for the concept of emotional styles see Reddy 2008) that are typical for the two departments.

In mixed focus groups, where participants did not represent a single team, they were generally more free to express criticism of their closest colleagues, including their superiors. One of the features of the obstetrics sector is that the superior of the neonatologists (chief doctor of the maternity hospital) is the obstetrician-gynaecologist, and these two professions are in conflicting relationships with each other, because they have different objects of care (the child and the woman in labour, respectively). A significant part of the reproaches of neonatologists is addressed to representatives of other levels of care and superiors, who are unable to hear the doctor's point of view, so he is 'ostracised' for his decisions:

> - Everyone tells you what to do, one said one thing, another one pointed out another thing, the third one advised the third thing. When you make a decision, it is already your responsibility, though. And this 'consilium' is no longer important, although, yes, you can write that you acted in agreement with someone, but the signature is yours and they will condemn you and your decision personally.
>
> - Although the decision has already been made, it is being discussed behind the back. For me, for example, the most difficult thing is that the team does not discuss everything directly with you, I mean they discuss and condemn you but they don't tell you anything at all. (A neonatologist at the maternity hospital, female, focus group materials, August 2023)

A stress area for doctors becomes the sole responsibility for medical decisions made and discussion of these decisions 'behind their backs', which creates an unhealthy atmosphere in the workplace and serves as a specific power management tool. Bosses (chief medical officers, heads of units) who are ready to hear alternative points of view and openly discuss mistakes, on the contrary, inspire trust and a desire to continue working in the team.

Maternity hospital nurses, as lower representatives of the medical hierarchy, complain even more actively about their superiors, that is, in their case, doctors in general:

> They [doctors] do not take the nurses' side, they do not protect them [. . .] and they can, for example, expose this publicly. There is a category of doctors, who listen to a mother's complaint, nod their head, take you to a corner and say that you were wrong, I mean you should have formulated or behaved differently, done something differently, but there are those, who begin to repeat what that mom said, in front of her and others, and go on telling you off, nagging. (A maternity hospital nurse, focus group materials, October 2023)

A nurse finds herself dependent both on the claims of mothers and on the authority of the doctor and thus feels most morally vulnerable in a situation where the doctor publicly reprimands her, thereby using her as a tool for solving problems with the child's mother. Nurses would like to receive protection and help from doctors, but in the end, the nurse, being at the bottom of the hierarchy, turns out to be 'always guilty'. At the same time, the nurses of the neonatal department here stand in solidarity with midwives, as equals in status and as those to whom it is customary to shift responsibility to. They complain of unjustified exploitation by doctors, which symbolically emphasises their low status:

> OK, let's take those surgeons. They come to your department and act as if, 'Everyone owes us, it's very important that you . . '. For example, I had a situation like that – there was a pack of sterile napkins, I put it next to him, opened it slightly, well, like that, that's it. We dressed him [in a sterile gown], and I went to another child. He is standing there, looking at me and saying, 'Can you give me a napkin?' Well, damn, you just need to reach out hand and pick it [but you ask me]. (A maternity hospital nurse, focus group materials, October 2023)

They also complain that doctors try to resolve issues using obscene language and shouting, as well as, among other things, their gender power:

> For example, they simply didn't talk to you, just sent you very far away and for a long time. For about ten minutes you are listening to all the swear words you know. And it's going on face to face, an adult man is standing right at you and yelling. It was very 'pleasant' every time. That's why I quit. (A maternity hospital nurse, focus group materials, October 2023)

Horizontal relationships in teams are described in terms of bullying and manipulation. The emotional intensity at work is so high that it even leads to fights. The only person capable of protecting nurses and building more acceptable relationships in the team becomes the 'head nurse, if she is "adequate", of course', too.

It is impossible to say exactly how true those stories really are, who actually bullied whom, how justified the doctor's anger was, and whether such symbolic violence of superiors over inferiors actually became the reason for dismissal or whether the focus group participant thus justified their dismissal in front of other participants. The only thing that can be stated is that the nurses actually used the focus group as a platform for speaking in the genre of complaints and lamentations (on the lamentation genre in Russian culture see Ries 1997), thereby signalling their difficult situation in the maternity sector, which they presented as dependent and powerless. It can be assumed that such a performance points to institutionally rooted problems that exist in the maternity sector, that is, lack of staff, exploitation of status in the hierarchy, lack of work standards for neonatal nurses, which they discussed separately. Perhaps this performance is a kind of cry for help, or a way to establish a relationship of solidarity with other participants. Almost no one talks about respectful relationships in the team, although it is possible that they are quite common in the experience of individual nurses.

So, as a rule, contradictions and emotionally tense relationships develop within one team between representatives of different levels of the emotional hierarchy. At the same time, a significant part of the difficulties arises at the intersection of different links and sectors of neonatal care.

When a patient moves from one level and sector of care to another, responsibility for him turns out to be socially distributed among specialists in these sectors. This creates the opportunity to rhetorically shift this responsibility to the previous link: neonatologists and nurses of the neonatal department of the maternity hospital blame obstetricians-gynaecologists for the child's condition (they use the term 'obstetric banditry'). Resuscitators and employees of the Department of Pathology of Prematurity are dissatisfied with both obstetricians-gynaecologists and neonatologists of the maternity hospital. Here is a fairly typical discussion of representatives of the subsequent sector addressed to primary care:

> - The maternity hospital staff is probably also not ready to work with them [children with extremely low body weight]. And they work so . . . let's put it this way . . . [carelessly].
>
> - Not as much as expected.
>
> - Not as much as we would like, right. And they have a feeling of uncertainty and some kind of fear that they will do something wrong, so they generally try not to do anything at all.
>
> - 'We didn't touch anything, didn't sanitise, didn't touch anything!' [maternity hospital staff say].
>
> - There he [a child] is lying and lying, thank God he's alive. This is also a little emotionally stressful. And yet, this is no longer in relation to patients, but more in relation to colleagues in maternity hospitals. They are also very different. We also have to constantly look for some common language with them. (RAC doctors, focus group materials, July 2023)

Doctors in the transport sector note the negligence of maternity hospital doctors, but at the same time, they try to save face, saying that they are actually simply afraid of such patients. The lack of competence of doctors creates a certain mistrust in their diagnosis and actions:

> - Yes. You don't trust anyone, you count child's fingers, examine the presence of everything, sort of a setup, a problem [congenital defects], and so on . . . even though ten people checked it before you. Every now and then it happens that a finger is missing, or something else, but no one noticed.
>
> - There may be a broken skull, and he is lying there for three days. You ask, 'What do you have here? The bone crunches'. (RAC doctors, focus group materials, July 2023)

In fact, doctors blame colleagues from other sectors for aggravating the patient's condition. Restraining emotions in such a situation and not directly expressing outrage is a significant part of the emotional work that doctors do at the intersection of sectors.

There is no confirmation that dissatisfaction with resuscitators and, in particular, employees of the transport resuscitation team arises due to the specifics of communication of the focus group, where the researchers were perceived as people close to the resuscitation and advisory service. Based on the materials received, it can be assumed that most of the accusations and grievances arise specifically against primary care employees, be they obstetricians-gynaecologists or neonatologists. Moreover, not only doctors but also nurses allow themselves this criticism:

> A nurse tells a story (apparently recent) that a child had a double pneumothorax, and then picked up sepsis, and was buried. The infection was passed on from his mother. Diaphragmatic hernia is a serious case. Sometimes if it is known in advance, the team is on duty waiting for the child. She is telling about a mother, who had been diagnosed with a streptococcal infection in her genitals, but the child was 'put into natural labour'. Naturally, he picked it up. Why didn't they do a caesarean section even though they'd known? They said that they didn't want the mother to have a stitch. 'What were you thinking about! They should have thought about the child!'. (The participant observation diary, ambulance, November 2023)

During the fieldwork, researchers were able to observe several situations of interaction between representatives of the maternity hospital and the transport team, which allowed them to conclude the structure of 'facework' and emotional work at the border of sectors.

> The transport team is busy with the child, but none of the maternity hospital doctors are visible. 'It seems to me that he is hot', says the doctor of the transport team, and the temperature begins to be measured. +38.1C. 'Have they overheated him?' The team members look at each other with displeasure, clearly understanding that the local doctors didn't pay attention, did something wrong, but this is not said directly. After some time, the head of the intensive

care unit of the maternity hospital comes into the ward and asks the team doctor for advice about another child in the ward. She begins to complain that she couldn't leave on time because the heavy babies began to be born, and there were two children with 'heart defects' and two twins. The team doctor says encouragingly, 'Alright, it's over, it's time to go home, we won't tell anyone!'. (the participant observation diary, maternity hospital, June 2023)

In this fragment, the transport team members non-verbally signal each other about the negligence of the maternity hospital doctors, and later, already in the ambulance, they will discuss this situation among themselves. However, they do not express this professional claim directly to their colleagues. On the contrary, dissatisfaction with the work of the maternity hospital staff is hidden, and the team doctor carries out emotional work to support a tired colleague. Such work on emotions allows them to maintain neutral or good relationships between personnel from different sectors, which facilitates work and helps to achieve informal agreements.

Here is another example of interaction between the team and maternity hospital staff:

A neonatologist meets us in the maternity hospital ward. She is a little fussy and friendly, she treats the transport team with some care and at some point, slips candy onto the gurney, which the incubator stands on. She says that the child is not hers at all, formally, the attending physician has left. In addition, in the room, a nurse says 'I will help you'. At the same time, she is often absent and she doesn't seem to strive to participate much, but you cannot say she doesn't do anything either. While working, a local nurse and members of the transport team are also discussing migrant children, 'whatever is happening in France, awaits us as well'. The maternity hospital doctor says that already thirty per cent of our births are 'non-Russian'. Then the team and maternity hospital doctors discuss the obstetricians, 'Oh, those paid childbirth, it happened because of the obstetricians'. Firstly, they 'caesared' her late and there was a long waterless period. Secondly, they did not pay attention to the infection and the mother's medical history, and did not tell the neonatologists. At some point, a local nurse complains that they were given two 'illegal immigrants'. (The participant observation diary, maternity hospital, July 2023)

In this fragment, the neonatologist is obviously happy about the arrival of the team, since there is a chance to shift responsibility for a difficult child onto them. She emphasises her favour both through communicative work and through a small gift that performs a contact-establishing function. In exchange, she gets the opportunity to leave work without staying longer than the official end time. Small talk, which is dedicated to migrants and 'ethnic' families, also fulfills its function of maintaining good relationships. On the one hand, this is also a professional conversation. There are the culprits – obstetricians and insufficiently examined mothers with non-Russian citisenship, who create medical and bureaucratic problems in all sectors of care. On the other hand, this conversation goes beyond the narrow professional area. It works with collective ideas and fears, characteristic of wider circles of ordinary people.

It is difficult to say to what extent all participants in the conversation actually share these ideas. But it is important to note that complaints, sweets, jokes, lowercase vocabulary, talking about the danger of migrants and other communication techniques are ways to maintain relationships and the work environment in situations of fatigue, uncertainty and nervous stress. That all creates a common communication field for the sake of more effective cooperation, especially taking into account that issues that are inconvenient for each other have to be settled bureaucratically. For example, in the last case, the team doctor eventually managed to 'lure' the curosurf drug, required for injection, from the maternity hospital doctor (this drug is only available in maternity hospitals) and insisted that the discharge include an infectious diagnosis, although this is an additional problem for the maternity hospital doctors related to registration with the epidemiological bureau. As a whole, such communication and emotional work pursue professional goals and put not only the staff's own comfort at the centre but also the benefit of the patient.

WORK AS A WAY OF LIFE

The previous section concludes with a story about how patients and their parents become part of the everyday, non-working lives of doctors and nurses. This section is devoted to how doctors draw boundaries between work and personal areas, and how they regulate their emotional world in connection with the peculiarities of their work.

As it was already mentioned, different sectors of neonatal care and teams have their own characteristics of emotional style, which are associated with institutional features, values, modes of management and so on in a particular organisation or in a particular department, the 'emotional practices' in them will be different. This will be demonstrated below, using the example of the way staff in different departments discuss emotions and experiences. First, the maternity hospital nurses say:

> Well, of course, there are such moments, especially at the end of the day. Well, it's been an intense day, the machines are screaming. Well, you can swear a bit in the morning, saying, who you are, what you are, where your things are. It seems to me that everyone is human. When you are tired, it still happens. . . . You have to throw it out somewhere, otherwise you will take it home, and then

> everyone at home will get it too. Therefore, perhaps, sometimes it is okay. (Maternity hospital nurse, focus group materials, October 2023)

> This greatly influences, when you come to work, when you are emotionally wound up and you really don't need anything else to bug and nag you, it's just. . . . It's not that you just did something wrong, it's just that you're somehow emotionally spread rot because you. . . . Well, you, well, are not like [they need]. . . . Here he is blond, and I am brunette, is it my bad? (Maternity hospital nurse, focus group materials, October 2023)

Maternity hospital nurses, during focus groups, emphasise the impossibility of restraining emotions in the workplace and the inability to completely 'leave' them at work. This, as can be seen from these quotes and from the material described in the previous sections, is due to their position in the hierarchy of the maternity hospital staff, which they perceive as vulnerable. However, a similar conversation about emotions, methods and limits of their expression is also typical for neonatologists of the maternity hospital:

> No, no, I don't try to cry during [work], but emotionally, for example, I can swear loudly enough. I mean I don't sit and cry, but when you don't agree, you try to prove your point of view and you are faced with complete misunderstanding and denial of, well, some absolutely obvious things [. . .]. And when you can't prove it and do it [your way], but later you turn out to be right, and no one says anything that you were right. . . . Well, I'm emotional in this regard. (A maternity hospital neonatologist, female, focus group materials, August 2023)

> Well, so you have to understand, in terms of the emotional state, it was some kind of difficult duty, and I left my work, okay, that's it, I'm going somewhere, I don't remember where exactly anymore. And I burst into tears because I missed the tram. Here, it's about emotional state. This is funny. I mean I was walking, but it had pulled out before I arrived. Catastrophe! I'm in hysterics. (A maternity hospital neonatologist, female, focus group materials, August 2023)

> Well, I'm just speaking from my experience. I have only been the head of the unit for a year; before that I wasn't. There are things that seem to finish me off personally, emotionally as well, because a person cannot come to work in a completely destabilised emotional state. [. . .] Such person cannot work properly, he cannot talk to anyone politely, he is simply emotionally exhausted. (A maternity hospital neonatologist, female, focus group materials, August 2023)

Crying in the workplace, especially in front of mothers and relatives, is postulated as an unacceptable manifestation of emotions. It must be taken outside the workspace, but manifestations of anger and the 'desire to fight' are quite acceptable. At the same time, doctors admit that due to fatigue and stress, they are in a 'destabilised' emotional state at work. As they are outside of work after a difficult duty, any 'non-medical' trigger can provoke a breakdown. The very words that people in this sector use to describe their emotional state and emotional culture as a whole are indicative – 'hysterical', 'throw out', 'emotionally spread rot', 'finish off', 'exhausted'. They have a vivid metaphorical basis and indicate the intensity of experiences or, in any case, how important it is for participants to present their emotional world in the focus group space.

Resuscitation doctors, both in the intensive care consulting service and in the intensive care unit, practically do not mention emotions in this way. Their world of experiences looks regulated, although not trouble-free. They talk about emotional culture in virtually professional terms.

> Of course, the problem [of the lack of psychological support] exists. I have been talking for a long time about the fact that a good psychological service should work in a department, [. . .] and psychologists should work in the same teams, closely cooperating with doctors, yes. I'm sure this is a service that can help us communicate with patients and ourselves. It is very important. Every person knows for himself, if he is tired, he cannot communicate normally. If he has some kind of resource, then this is a completely different quality of communication. (An intensive care unit doctor, male, focus group materials, August 2023)

> There was a moment, when we had pneumothoraxes one after another. When an emergency occurs, a child's lung ruptures, most often this is accompanied by a fairly progressive deterioration in the child's condition. Well, naturally, you need to do everything quickly. It all depends on the coordinated work of the whole team, your team, the maternity hospital staff, and something else. But when we had them in a row, then it was probably already the third or fourth pneumothorax, then it looked for me [as usual] as inserting a peripheral catheter. There were no emotions anymore. (an RAC doctor, female, focus group materials, July 2023)

In these quotes, doctors talk calmly in terms of professionalising emotions about emergency or exhausting work situations and the need for psychological help in controlling their own emotional state.

> Well, just keep in mind that burnout still exists. Now, although our ladies say that this is a minor point, I disagree. It certainly exists, it is present, and so on, but it is removed, relieved in different ways, unfortunately. If we take, so to speak, well, I mean, my colleagues, mostly male, you can't imagine how many are already dead, you see they are no longer alive, and I started working with them. Do you know how many have switched to using all sorts of psychoactive substances? This is something that, so to speak, has a very strong impact on. . . . So this side of burnout certainly exists, of course. (An RAC doctor, male, focus group materials, July 2023)

> [On the one hand], you have this ability to nod and look into the eyes compassionately, but simultaneously not really perceive at all. But this is an ideal model, this does not happen. Most doctors, one way or another, they try this situation on themselves, whether they want it or not, and this leads gradually, year after year, to burnout, post-traumatic stress disorder, and everything else. There are such things there, insomnia, a bunch of other things, I don't know. (An intensive care unit doctor, male, focus group materials, August 2023)

In these fragments, the interlocutors talk about the emotional state in psychological, medical, and psychiatric terms (burnout, substance use, insomnia, post-traumatic stress disorder) or in terms of medical ethics and deontology (compassion), thereby emphasising their professional approach to the world of emotions.

In the neonatal pathology department, there is a third, in some sense, intermediate version of talking about emotions at work:

> When I started working, for the first five years, it was very difficult for me in various ways. I mean I was unable to talk quietly, I broke down and shouted. I could scream at my husband, at my mother, at my eldest child. [It happened] just out of the blue. [The husband] one day said, 'Either you pull yourself together and control yourself, or we're breaking up'. [Now] there is no such emotional component anymore. But at first, it was very strong, and my loved ones suffered greatly from this, to such an extent that, [for example], my husband says, 'We are sometimes even so afraid of you that when you come home, we all hide in the corners.' I didn't lash out here [at work], I lashed out at my loved ones. And he pointed this out to me, it was very unpleasant to listen to that, because it seemed to me that there was no such thing he was talking about, that they were all fools, I was just pointing out their shortcomings. This was not the case. Well, then it dawned on me, since I'm already quite adult, wise, and now I'm somehow more relaxed about it. But when two or three years ago a girl I was taking care of died, she died in intensive care, but, nevertheless, she got worse here, then I was knocked out for about . . . six months exactly, I couldn't get over and come to my senses for a long time, I even went to a psychologist, because I couldn't put up with that and accept that in myself, that kind of thing. (A doctor of the neonatal pathology department, female, focus group materials, September 2023)

The mentioned 'breakdowns', which are impossible at work, are transferred to the home space. At the same time, the doctor talks about her condition in terms of the gradual professionalisation of emotions, detachment from them and the gradual acquisition of self-control. In order to do all this work on herself, she turns to a specialist psychologist, that is, she actually seeks professional support to regulate her own experiences related to her line of work.

As noted at the very beginning of the chapter, in general, all interlocutors tend to use the term 'professional/emotional burnout' in one way or another in relation to their work in general or their condition in particular. It is impossible to make an accurate conclusion about whether the participants in the study actually have burnout. Even if they themselves talk about it, it is impossible to say what factors provoked it. This is the task of a psychologist. In this case, it is only possible to note some correlations that the interlocutors themselves draw between emotional stress and the conditions, which it is associated with.

As can be seen from the quotes above, employees of intensive care units of the hospital and transport sector talk about burnout, but at the same time they seem to alienate these conditions from themselves, and none of them applies this term to themselves. In the intensive care unit, they describe their own state at work rather in terms of passion, interest in work and 'burning'. 'It's like solving a complex math problem,' says an RAC doctor about his work in the ambulance. 'We are all adrenaline junkies!' jokes the intensive care unit doctor. 'Workaholics!' echoes another. 'Interesting, not boring, absolutely not boring,' says the nurse of this department. Work in both intensive care and emergency rooms is described in terms of the only possible life choice. 'In intensive care, you understand that you either have to work in this field for the rest of your days, or radically change something, leave it and learn something completely different, I don't know, it might be, [. . .] dentistry, ultrasound or any mortal thing, but be away from all this. The ambulance is a way of life,' says the RAC nurse. Another one is turning to the researcher, while getting out of the ambulance, and says, 'Try to feel how important it is to be on earth,' thereby making it clear how much the work has literally become ingrained and built into the body. In such a structure, when professional life and identity are closely connected, dismissal or leaving the profession is almost impossible, because in essence, if a person continues to remain in it, then he lives 'on adrenaline' and is not in danger of burnout.

The only complaint about the working conditions of ambulance workers remains a complaint about back problems, which are caused by deficiencies in the infrastructure, such as uncomfortable chairs in the ambulance, ill-designed ramps for incubators. Only one of the intensive care unit nurses, citing a difficult work schedule, admits, 'I'm one hundred per cent burnt out'. However, due to life circumstances, she cannot quit because she needs to provide for her family, and the intensive schedule is her own choice. Thus, she connects her burnout not with the specifics of working with patients itself, but with fatigue from her own life circumstances.

In the neonatal pathology department, they talk about burnout rather in terms of fatigue in specific, institutionally determined situations, that is, a long absence of vacation, for example, or a large number of patients.

> Well, of course, there's a huge difference, when you control ten children and when you look after fourteen or fifteen. This means that you can knock off earlier, at 5 p.m. or you have to stay until 8 p.m. (A doctor of the neonatal pathology department, female, focus group materials, September 2023)

Thus, burnout is described rather as a temporary condition that is not related to ideas about one's own professional applicability and does not affect the understanding of professional identity, which also turns out to be important for the doctors of this department:

> Write in your book that the most interesting thing is to work at the second stage! What is interesting in the maternity hospital, what is there? You gave birth, transferred, the intensive care unit is also there, so you extubated, intubated, that's all. Yes, and the resuscitation and advisory service delivered [a child] (laughing). It's us, who gets sweets! (A doctor of the neonatal pathology department, female, focus group materials, September 2023)

In this fragment, doctors contrast themselves with the 'adrenaline' work of resuscitators, who are surrounded by a heroic aura, and declare that their professional direction is no less valuable and working in the neonatal pathology department is no less exciting.

In the maternity hospital sector, stories about burnout take on a more systemic and pronounced tone, they are more personal. Here's what nurses say about it:

> - I'm burned out. Well, I just realised that these two job shifts are the last ones, they got me down very completely, because of this doctor's attitude, which was [hard] for me [. . .]. I actually quit because I had a nervous breakdown right on the street after a shift of mine. I mean I went out, I couldn't call a taxi, it wasn't coming to me, it was raining for forty minutes, I was sitting on a bench and crying, then I realised that I couldn't stand it, go on like this anymore, it was very difficult for me. I quit and found another job. For the first six months there, it seems to me that I was just getting over, because in general there was no such active work there, I just went there and thought, 'Wow, it's good, so great!' And then I realised that I couldn't do it anymore. Well, I really couldn't, I didn't enjoy what I did. Before that, I'd been really passionate about my work, I'd thought, 'Damn, it's so great, these are children, I'm helping. I like it'. And now I just go to work day by day as if operating a lathe. But I didn't like that kind of attitude to work. So I decided that it was probably time to end that, because I seemed to be doing no harm, but I wasn't doing much good either.
>
> - Probably, sometimes this happens to everyone, when you come home from work and think, 'Lord, I want to sell herring somewhere at the market', so that you can stand and you, and if someone pisses you off, slap him with this

> a herring right in the face. This happens. Although, it seems to me, more often people think like this, 'Lord, I'm so tired of all this, I'll go put stamps or sell herring'. (Maternity hospital nurses, focus group materials, October 2023)

On the one hand, professional burnout turns out to be associated with the attitude of superior specialists towards subordinates and a low place in the hierarchy, that is, with the institutional structure and emotional culture of specific organisations. On the other hand, it is important to note that the connection between specialisation and identity turns out to be less close here, that is, nurses shuttle between the department of physiology and the resuscitation unit, change institutions, and if they see value in their profession as a whole ('helping children'), then a specific piece of medical care does not become a 'way of life' for them.

Maternity hospital doctors also talk about burnout in terms of institutional conditions, but they are quite different:

> Yes, I work for myself. [Just imagine that] I got sick. Can you imagine? I worked for myself, too. As I get sick, nobody cares about that – either the country or the people. . . . Nobody needs me. [. . .] You feel left off. Although you have worked in medicine all your life, and you have dedicated your whole life to this, you like it, it is organic to you, it is yours, you came and work by vocation, you did not imagine yourself in anything else, but [at this moment no one cares]. Now, the more I look around, the more I understand that you can break out [of this vicious circle], you can live a different life, experience different situations. In my opinion, this is not good, it is wrong. This is probably what professional burnout is all about. It's important to understand what you're putting into it now, because you've put yourself into this work completely, and people know how I work, and you understand how much you've already put in it, because you needed it, but no one else did. (A maternity hospital neonatologist, female, focus group materials, August 2023)

> It seems to me that in our country, well, I don't know, at least at that stage of development, well, let's be honest [. . .]. Some period of time passes, and you realise that it's over, you're tired. You can't stand it anymore, no way. I think there was some moment, when [. . .] we realised that we were faced with this. COVID has finally finished us off. You all had professional burnout, and that was the end of us. [. . .] I believe that we devote a lot of time to [work], a lot of energy, a lot of our emotions, and even, in principle, [our] lives in general. [. . .] So we have to make up for [the loss of strength] from somewhere a little, and have to find where to take it from. When COVID started, stories were getting around that they would pass such a law, and I'm sure it's the only solution that could cure some doctors from professional burnout, i.e. [the law] if a person has worked for fifteen years in medicine, he has the right to take a year off, say, with fifty per cent compensation of his or her salary. Then the person could reach closure and take a breath. Our system, though, essentially forces the person to quit,

when he can't toil away at work anymore. (A maternity hospital neonatologist, female, focus group materials, August 2023)

Doctors make themselves clear that burnout affects all workers in the sector. Those who deny it aren't simply telling the truth. In their rhetoric, burnout is closely associated with total institutional insecurity, on the one hand, and, on the other hand, with an extreme degree of uncertainty. They see significant life meaning and value in their profession, but, like maternity hospital nurses, they are more flexible in their choice of place of work and are not so tied to their narrow specialisation. They are ready to try something new. At the same time, they do not fully see and sense the evaluation and appreciation of their work by the state in particular.

It's worth noting that a common thread across all care sectors is the conversation around the structure of boundaries between work and personal time and space. It turns out that despite attempts to get rid of thoughts about work and avoid bringing them home, very few healthcare professionals succeed in doing so. 'Yes, [I wish I could say so] I turned off the lathe and left, then came back in the morning, turned it on again, and began to turn the piece of iron. This is not true at all, though,' says a hospital's resuscitator. At the same time, the metaphor of the production line at the factory is indicative, because in the quote above, the maternity hospital nurse talks about her burnout in precisely the same terms, 'I just go to work day by day as if operating a lathe'. This means that treating work as an assembly line production that can be forgotten outside the walls of the medical institution is not encouraged within the framework of corporate medical culture, because it signals excessive detachment, disengagement and burnout of the medical specialist.

> Frameworks can save someone, but for me it doesn't work. For example, until I make sure, I mean until it is confirmed one, two, three times that everything has settled down for the child, his condition is okay . . . until that moment I cannot calm down, have a calm life. No framework helps. My mother was [a doctor] and always . . . when she defended me from someone, she always used to say 'they are living children, they are not pears, they are not nails or boxes'. That's probably true. (A maternity hospital neonatologist, female, focus group materials, August 2023)

> Well, you can't forget everything at all. If something has upset you so much, well, you can't come home and say, 'It's a wonderful world! Let's dance!' No matter whether you want it or not, if something [has hurt you] a lot, or on the contrary, something very good [has happened], you want to share it with everyone. For example, I want to tell everyone about how they [children and parents] gave me flowers, and I really wanted to [share that]. Or, on the contrary, someone upset you, like this situation with twins [when the mother came to see

> only the healthy child and ignored the second one with Down syndrome. Later she abandoned him]. And you merely come back home to talk calmly. Nothing of the kind, you can't say, 'Oh, we treated [a child] there today, we cut off this and that for him'. No, they won't understand me at all. No one is a doctor in my family, [. . .] I will scare them, [. . .] these are all strong experiences. Of course, any person, no matter where he works, also brings his worries and experiences home. (A doctor of the neonatal pathology department, female, focus group materials, September 2023)

I can't speak for others, how it happens for them, how people unwind. For example, when I manage to be alone, I still continue to think, 'If such a test comes tomorrow, what kind of medicine will I prescribe then?' Or, it happens when I swim [in the pool] in the evenings. While swimming, I'm thinking, counting the doses of antibiotics. I swam one lane, there, counted it for one, another lane – for another patient. . . . That's the way it is. Unfortunately, yes, there is no escape from this. (An intensive care unit doctor, male, focus group materials, August 2023)

> [Sounds} of the monitors are beeping in your ears all the time. Once I came to my parents after many shifts, I had several days off. I remember I was sleeping, and when my mother woke me up, I said, 'Mom, turn off the monitor, it's beeping very loudly, I can't sleep tight'. Well, I mean they [work moments] spin and spin and spin right in your brain, especially when often [difficult situations arise]. That kind of thing. (A maternity hospital nurse, focus group materials, October 2023)

Workspace and time break into the personal and home life during conversations with relatives, especially if they are doctors. They manifest themselves in the form of emotional experiences and 'breakdowns', worries about the patient's condition, professional thoughts about how to prescribe medications or what therapeutic tactics to choose, or even simply in the form of sensory experiences, as in the case of the sounds of the monitor, which seemed to be absorbed into the body, or back pain from heavy incubators. On the one hand, the seepage of work into everyday life does not allow the staff to rest and relax, take a breath, or unwind. On the other hand, this is clear evidence of its high symbolic significance because healing and saving children is a mission deeply embedded in their own identity.

CONCLUSION

A careful look at the history of medicine helps to notice a steady increase in the number of medical specialities. This differentiation has led to the fact that the general term ‘doctor’ without indicating specialisation can tell little about the activities of a person in this profession. Gone are the days of universalism, when a doctor was a general specialist and provided medical care to patients of all age groups, regardless of nosology and various forms of the disease. Nowadays, some doctors may not interact with patients at all, describing images or samples of tissues and cells, others are engaged in disease prevention and healthy nutrition, and others are engaged in aesthetic medicine. This differentiation gradually formed an idea about medical specialities with high and low levels of responsibility (Carroll and Buddenbaum 2013), where the main criterion for the degree of responsibility is the severity of the consequences arising from medical errors or malpractice.

Specialities with a high risk of liability usually include representatives of emergency medicine (emergency doctors, resuscitators), surgeons, obstetricians and radiologists. Neonatologists, working in intensive care units, daily face critical situations that require them to have a certain level of stress tolerance. The causes of stress can be different. These may be the risks of criminal prosecution (Korobeev and Shirshov 2020), moral responsibility for decision-making within their official duties (Deligianni et al. 2023), communication with parents of seriously ill patients, interaction with colleagues and so on. Raising the issue of the emotional dimension in the work of a neonatologist, like any other specialist with a high risk of liability, it is difficult to formulate a clear research plan and distinguish between different layers of emotional experiences, such as attitude towards the patient, self-reflection or emotions associated with professional risks.

On the one hand, legal and bureaucratic aspects can significantly influence the attitude towards the patient, as, for example, was noted in the history of the development of neonatology and the provision of care to early preterm infants at the formation stage of the neonatal service. On the other hand, in addition to the legal perspective, there is a professional view of the problem, determined by technological capabilities. Today, technology makes it possible to care for newborns who were doomed several decades ago. Meanwhile, expanding the boundaries of technological capabilities inevitably creates new problem groups. If today children older than 26 weeks of gestation have relatively favourable prospects, then in the group of children aged 22 to 25 weeks, the results are not so encouraging (Torchin, Morgan and Ancel 2020). This also applies to children who have suffered severe asphyxia or newborns with severe congenital pathology. Technologies and the professional actions of doctors make it possible to maintain the lives of those patients for a long time, but this work has its own emotional price, which not only the parents of those patients but also doctors have to pay. Given the fact that the result of the work largely depends on the degree of material security, staffing, and the degree of professional organisation of the treatment process in each particular institution, then it becomes clear how differently the work of a neonatologist can be perceived in terms of emotional experiences in different sectors of neonatal care.

Thus, this chapter examined, on the one hand, the emotional accompaniment of forming a patient from a newborn, and on the other, the value dimension of the work of those actors who actually participate in the process of 'birth' of this patient.

Hence, the degree of opacity, incomprehensibility of the child's condition, and the unpredictability of the dynamics of this condition play an important role for doctors in their attitude towards the patient and in assessing their own emotional and cognitive involvement in working with him. This uncertainty and incomprehensibility of the patient's condition may be associated with various previous circumstances. For example, for primary care, this is a new patient who has just been born and does not yet have a medical history. For subsequent stages, it is a maternity hospital or hospital treatment in another city, which contributes to the history of previous links of care and plays a significant role. Shortcomings in diagnosis and prescriptions at the previous stages can sort of 'obscure' the patient, making him 'a pig in a poke', according to the interlocutors. In situations of such uncertainty, medical decision-making is complicated, which significantly increases the burden on the doctor.

It is important to underline that emotions in the discourse of physicians are more closely related to professional decisions. In fact, when talking about emotions towards a child patient, they talk about the level of tension in this situation and the degree of their own cognitive involvement in the process of rescue or treatment. Moreover, even if a child is endowed with some personal traits and social characteristics, this happens either in line with typified cultural patterns (attribution of gender stereotypes, an increase in the amount of baby talk with the growth of the baby's activity, etc.), or in accordance with professional interest (e.g., a doctor is more interested in working with premature babies than with full-term ones suffering from the consequences of asphyxia. Or a nurse feels uncomfortable dressing a child with an atypically developed body). At the same time, evaluative judgements and emotions are caused by the therapeutic situation itself and not by the patient himself. Despite all the emotional, evaluative and communicative reactions that arise in the process of interaction with the child, he or she is still not considered a separate person who is in any way responsible for his or her behaviour.

At the same time, the category of responsibility permeates the interaction under study. Thus, a therapeutic situation, which is subject not only to professional but, as it turns out, also to moral assessment, may be determined by circumstances that make it difficult, urgent or incomprehensible. In the discourse of doctors, responsibility for the patient's condition is assigned to the actors who were involved in his or her life at all previous stages. They can be reproductive doctors, who advised the mother to make another attempt at IVF after several unsuccessful attempts, or gynaecologists, who dissuaded her from having an abortion, although there were medical indications for it; or the mother herself, who decided to keep the child with a known pathology or was not examined enough during pregnancy; or obstetricians, who incorrectly delivered the child; or primary care doctors, who were incompetent or could not correctly diagnose the child in a maternity hospital.

Hence, parents and colleagues from other sectors/levels of care are those persons who evoke the most of personally oriented emotions. While 'practicing' emotions (Scheer, ibid) the doctors have to work with their performance somehow; that is, communicate according to corporate and cultural norms, regulate and contain, name them in order to make them more accountable, mobilise publicly to construct their own professional identity. Interactions with colleagues and parents are areas of greatest tension, where much of the visible emotional work takes place (see Scheer, Hochschild, ibid), although the extent of this interaction varies across different sectors of care and across different health professions (physicians, nursing staff).

For instance, the emotions of a mother can interfere with doctors, take away strength and cause irritation, since sympathy is difficult to express due to professional detachment. If the parent is not in any way part of the 'extended' patient, as it was described in the case of the resuscitation and transport unit, then irritation and inattention to the parent's emotions can manifest itself, and emotional control (work) weakens. In those links where the parent plays a more significant role, where she is expected to understand, at least to some extent, what is happening with her child and, thereby, help doctors do their job, in those circumstances seeking contact and emotionally acceptable forms of communication with parents becomes a more important task. Direct interaction between colleagues from different sectors, communication is usually based more on restraining emotions; that is, discussion of wrong decisions, criticism, expression of dissatisfaction, irritation or anger is transferred to their own team with the pragmatic goal of maintaining long-term loyal relationships with colleagues from another sector. Such corporate emotional tactics help to reduce tension at the border between the maternity hospital – RAC transport service and transport service – paediatric hospital sectors, which makes it possible to more successfully solve practical problems for the benefit of the patient. At the same time, in the absence of direct interaction between sectors, emotional work becomes secondary, giving way to professional criticism.

Interactions within a team can also serve as a source of emotional tension, but if this were articulated for researchers (it seems to be not entirely ethical to discuss one's own team in a focus group), then this mainly concerned vertical, hierarchical relationships. Thus, nurses can criticise doctors, managers can criticise older nurses, doctors can criticise higher managers (chief nurses, heads of units) and so on. The reason for criticism, in many respects, also becomes the nature of the distribution and imputation of responsibility for professional actions and decisions within the team.

At the same time, apparently, different medical teams are characterised by different emotional styles (Reddy, ibid) and different ways of building both horizontal and vertical relationships. Different sectors of health care have different institutional conditions, such as wages and workload levels. One of the objectives of this part, as formulated at the beginning, was to look at how relevant it is for doctors to understand their own emotional and professional burnout. As the results of the study showed, the interlocutors attributed this largely to the nature of relationships in the team and the peculiarities of institutional conditions, and not to the specifics of the work itself.

However, both the nature of the work and the patient have their own specifics regarding emotional stress. Returning to the conversation about the important value of professionalism and making medically correct decisions, as well as responsibility, it is necessary to point out that each doctor ultimately bears personal responsibility, no matter what attempts he or she makes in order to rhetorically shift responsibility for the patient's condition onto someone else or change its configuration. This maximises the emotional burden on him or her, especially taking into account that the work of medical personnel in the studied levels of care is associated with a high probability of death or disability of the patient, with actions and decision-making in emergency conditions. Paradoxically, it is precisely work in the most extreme conditions, according to the rhetoric of doctors, that seems to be least associated with burnout. Thus, the study shows that, first of all, it is emergency resuscitation and intensive care unit doctors who evaluate their work as a 'way of life', most tightly integrating a narrow professional identity into the construction of their personality.

Actually, the possibility of the patient's death and the prospect of his or her long dying also become a difficult component of the work, requiring internal regulation of emotions and state. Working with palliative children is deemed to be an activity that takes energy, time and emotional and economic resources. In fact, palliative care, one might say, to some extent, profanes and calls into question the central meanings of the work of a doctor of neonatology specialisation; that is, instead of a struggle for life, it becomes an accompaniment to death. In this conversation, another responsible actor appears, and it is the state and in particular the sphere of legislative decisions in the field of reproduction and neonatal care. A palliative, 'unpromising' child is actually considered the area of responsibility of other sectors, professions and types of activity, such as hospices, children's homes and volunteer organisations. It is there that working with such a patient again takes on its deep meaning.

NOTES

1. The term 'foetus', which was heard in other sectors of neonatal care, was not used for this category of children. Maternity hospital doctors might not have used generally accepted jargon and labels due to a lack of practice, working with those children (the focus groups were mainly attended by representatives of maternity hospitals, where children with extremely low body weight were rarely born). Also, this might have been due to the incorrectness of public use of such a term.
2. It is worth noting that the nurse's remarks focus on physiological manifestations, apparently not only because they are clinically significant but because she deals with basic care in her work.
3. Institutionally, the resuscitation team of the transportation service, often referred to as such in this chapter, is the part of RAC.
4. A popular food and goods delivery service in Russia.

Chapter 5

Managerial, Economic and Political Entities of a Newborn

INTRODUCTION

The first chapter of this book showed how medical practices and organisational conditions for providing neonatal care and, subsequently, the very legal status of a newborn are changing due to professional initiatives. However, the work of health professionals and organisations that provide newborn care is currently highly dependent on formal and bureaucratic rules, including regulatory frameworks and law enforcement practices. In general, the fairly strong bureaucratic regulation of medical practice in Russia (and earlier in the USSR (Field 1953)) is usually described as an integral part and important characteristic of this healthcare system (Mansurov and Yurchenko 2004; Litvina et al. 2019). In this context, the 'managerial logic of regulation' (Freidson 2001) largely dominates both the market and professional logics (Borozdina & Novkunskaya 2022) and consequently limits the professional autonomy of doctors and nursing staff (Borozdina 2018, 2023). This study aims to contribute to this debate and look at how formal rules and standards, legal frameworks and law enforcement, among others, influence the fate of newborn patients, that is, their legal and civil status, their 'patient careers' (Goffman 1959) within institutionalised health care, and even their symbolic or political status outside the medical context.

This chapter shows how, in the field under study, the current system of financing and regulation of health care, as well as the contradictions in this field, influence the trajectory of hospitalisation, diagnosis and treatment of newborn patients who require critical care. Referring to observational data, interviews and focus groups, it reconstructs how the newborn is presented in a variety of interaction and communication situations as a 'unit of account' or 'legal exposure'. This can manifest itself both in decisions to admit the patient to a particular institution if there is a free ‘bed’ to be taken there and, conversely, in the symbolic ‘assignment’ of social and cultural statuses to him or her, but for the sole purpose of freeing up a bed.

Thus, we plan to consider in more detail those social situations where a newborn is presented primarily as a set of economic and legal categories that are diligently counted, measured and distributed among different organisations. In doing so, we try, on the one hand, to show the inconsistency of the legal and economic fields, in which neonatal care is provided. On the other hand, however, there is an attempt to conceptualise these dimensions of neonatal care and show that the newborn patient has not only a physical body with a certain clinical condition and social statuses but also bureaucratic, legal and even economic entities.

The first section of the chapter describes how the ‘bureaucratic body’ of a newborn patient is formed, that is, his or her documented history, which in certain contexts turns out to be the main determinant of his or her further trajectory of (de)hospitalisation, as well as how it is created in multiple situations of negotiations between different medical professionals working as representatives of different medical institutions. It, in particular, will address how the ‘paper body’ can be ‘born’ even before a patient’s actual birth and how it can remain in the system of medical communications much longer than he or she does (both after discharge and, in some cases, after death).

It is shown further that the formation of such a documentary biography of a newborn patient occurs not only within the framework of his clinical history. This process reflects the complex system of distribution of material and intangible resources that constitute the essence of the work of the neonatal care service. This study also analyses the resources that are key for the work of neonatologists, nurses and healthcare managers, how they are distributed in this field, and what communication features cause a shortage to occur. In particular, it describes how the funding system and the lack of material resources in neonatology lead to the need to constantly adapt imperfect infrastructure to clinical tasks and also affect clinical decisions regarding the treatment and monitoring of a newborn patient.

It then examines how the broader political context indirectly, but still significantly, influences the organisation and implementation of newborn care. The political ‘entity’ in particular is manifested in the additional symbolic status of newborns, who turn out to be not only long-awaited children for their relatives and a care recipient for medical professionals but also a key indicator of the work of regional governors. This symbolic burden on each newborn creates additional dimensions of control both within and between medical organisations and professional communities, as well as in the broader sociopolitical context. The downside of such multiple control is the responsibility for clinical and routing decisions made. It is distributed unevenly in the context of negotiations between different professionals and organisations, and sometimes this distribution resembles a game of 'hot potato'.

The legal context is a separate dimension of control that is relevant to our field of study. The inconsistency of legal regulation and law enforcement in the field of medical care in Russia constantly emerged as significant topics in the analysis of the empirical data, and legal exposure for incorrectly completed medical documentation reminded researchers that this was a constant component of the work of medical professionals, providing neonatal care. In this context, a newborn and his/her 'paper body' take on yet another additional entity of legal risks and potential administrative or criminal sanctions. In order to ensure the safety of the participants in the study, the empirical illustrations for this section mainly are media publications on the most high-profile legal cases in the field of medical care for newborns, which were also mentioned by the informants in interviews and during observations.

The final section of the chapter is dedicated to those newborn patients who are 'on the margins' or even in the grey areas of all those bureaucratic, financial, political and legal contexts. This part examines the formation of the 'paper body' and the trajectory of the (de)hospitalisation of patients, who were physically born into the field under study but legally not well integrated into it. First, these empirical stories reveal that 'blind spots', like niches of uncertainty and contradictions that medical professionals have to resolve manually, are still present in this area, despite the highly bureaucratic nature of the medical care system and multiple controls over the work of medical professionals. Secondly, the stories of such patients show that, in addition to the analysed entities/identities, broader 'cultural' entities, associated with ethnic and religious traditions (or ideas about them), can be intentionally constructed for them.

A PATIENT AS A UNIT OF ACCOUNT

> A person in modern culture exists insofar as he or she is recorded and presented in various kinds of documents. (Baiburin 2017: 9)

We, as researchers tried to get as close as possible to the direct experience of neonatologists, nurses and other research participants in the field of neonatal care in observations and interviews during fieldwork. Given the methodological limitations associated with both autoethnographic data and biases, and those created by external observers, we tried to describe the direct professional practices of doctors and nurses and unprovoked communication situations in as much detail as possible. These data revealed many additional dimensions of assessment of a newborn patient in the field under study. As shown in previous chapters, a newborn patient possesses not only a body (which health professionals objectify and medicalise in great detail), but also social statuses associated with his or her gender, ethnicity, family economic class and other characteristics. It was also emphasised (see chapter 3) that some of these statuses were predetermined by the formal rules of medical care and the way it was financed and organised. These contexts of a newborn's 'patient career' (Goffman 1959) remain largely invisible to his family and outside observers, but they have an equally significant influence on his or her fate. Here is how one of the informants describes them:

> The thing is that any fact of providing medical service begins and ends for the uninitiated people exclusively with clinical care, with the need for a correct diagnosis, timely prescription of laboratory and interpretative tests, and correct treatment here and now. [But] a very important point, of course, is initially correctly planned routing. Be it from home, from a maternity hospital, from another medical institution, from the street, whichever. So, this is absolutely teamwork, where correct and timely decisions and their practical implementation must be made here and now. This is truly a multi-level process that . . . Just as the rules of the road are written on someone's corpses, the rules of our medical care are written, unfortunately, in the opposite way, too. And it must be constantly analysed. This is done by skilful professionals. Laws are written, amendments to laws are issued, and, indeed, this is very important work. Thus, in parallel with the transition of our healthcare to a monetary basis, and this became possible only after the transition to a system of mandatory health insurance, the need arose to create certain departments in almost all medical institutions, regardless of the form of ownership in them – either private or state, a federal institution on budget financing or an ordinary city clinic. I mean the need arose to create such offices, which began, not from a good life, to gradually grow, and which were engaged, say, in legal and financial support for the healthcare provision. (An interview with the deputy chief physician for administrative and expert work, October 2023)

The extensive quotation above touches upon several issues that are significant for subsequent analysis. Firstly, it turns out to be inseparably linked simultaneously to several different dimensions of the work of the neonatal service, that is, clinical, organisational, legislative and financial. Secondly, the informant highlights the growing influence of financial and legal support for neonatological care, reflected, among other things, in the complex organisational structure. And, thirdly, the existing system of rules (both formal and informal) is defined not as an isolated and 'external' phenomenon to medical work, but as a direct consequence of clinical decisions and their results as well as the conditions that shape them.

This section details these complex interweavings of bureaucratic, financial and infrastructural dimensions of neonatal care and attempts to trace how they are translated into the practices of doctors and nurses and the trajectories of newborn patients.

The epigraph to this section is a quote from Albert Baiburin's book on the Soviet passport. The idea behind it may seem maximalist to the reader, but in some contexts it reflects the high symbolic significance of documents, which can simultaneously be considered the material embodiment of state management and control (Hull 2008), as well as forms structuring social interactions in medicine (Berg 1996). The empirical field under study is shaped by two such contexts at least – the bureaucratic institutions of post-Soviet Russia, partially inherited from the Soviet era (Baiburin 2017), and the peculiarity of medical organisations, in which diagnoses and their documentation can historically be considered as entities, embodying diagnostic and therapeutic practices and social expectations regarding various diseases and their treatments (Rosenberg 2002).

The patient's documentation can be seen in these multiple bureaucratic contexts as another entity of a newborn patient. One of the previous studies proposed the concept of a 'paper patient', as a set of medical communications and decisions, mediated and embodied exclusively in the form of documents (Klepikova et al. 2023). In turn, this idea was borrowed from Nikita Shevchenko, who is engaged in another research plot, the so-called 'paper conscript' (2023). In both cases, a patient's medical history and a conscript's personal file were studied as a bureaucratic or pre-documentary 'self' (file-self), that is, an image of a person, embodied in documents and created by various actors in accordance with both normative rules and informal ways of circumventing them (Baiburin 2017; Fitzpatrick 2005).

Our empirical analysis further provides multiple practical examples of newborn patients' 'paper body' formation and the likely influence of the created medical history on their further routing and treatment. Analytically, it continues the tradition of the anthropology of bureaucracy in medicine and examines existing evidence as both a constitutive element of medical practice (Berg 1996) and an organisational infrastructure enabling the coordination of different contexts (Berg and Bowker 1997).

'Paper Body'

> We put a child in the car, I fill in his medical card and we leave. After 30 minutes, on the road, approaching the entrance to the children's hospital, I open the folder with documents and realise I'd forgot all the transfer papers (extract, parental consents, and photocopies of documents) [. . .]. We discuss how we will be scolded in the hospital. I call my colleague [from another RAC team], and she says she took the documents [. . .]. There is no doctor at the post. I immediately turn to the nurse, 'You're going to tell us off now, I apologise in

advance, but we forgot all the documents in the maternity hospital . . . we didn't forget the child, though!' She says [with surprise], 'How come? All the documents!?' (Participant observation diary, RAC unit, children' hospital, January 2020)

This rather ironic fragment of an autoethnographic diary clearly shows that various kinds of a child's documents (both medical and social, such as compulsory medical insurance policy, personal insurance policy number, parents' passport details and birth certificate) are as significant component of routing for the work of doctors and nurses and treatment as the child himself. The puzzled exclamation of the nurse in the dialogue with the doctor of the resuscitation and advisory service shows how much the lack of necessary documents can complicate her work (and the work of the whole department). The results of observations and focus group data indicate that the collection, completion and compilation of documents in terms of time and labour costs sometimes exceed the actual clinical work. As described in the previous chapter, it is bureaucratic work that sometimes reduces satisfaction from the profession and even leads to emotional burnout. However, this is one component that cannot be avoided. Moreover, the preparation of a child's documentary history can begin in some cases even before his or her birth (e.g., in the case of diseases and pathologies diagnosed in utero):

Natalya [head of the neonatal department in X maternity hospital] calls at about 11 o'clock and says they are planning a cesarean section in the X-maternity hospital. There is a child with congenital hydrothorax (fluid in the pleural cavity) there. Since I don't know what condition the child will be born in, I call the therapist and ask him if there are free nitric oxide reducers in the department [. . .]. We are going to the X-maternity hospital. At the maternity hospital we are greeted with joy, 'You've arrived so quickly'. In the ward at this time, nurses are placing a peripheral venous catheter. The head of the unit says they should take an X-ray picture now. She's also surprised that we've arrived so quickly. I am examining the child. The radiologist arrives and takes a picture. The head of the neonatology department of the maternity hospital brings me an ultrasound report from the medical genetic centre [done during pregnancy]. There is no checkout yet, because we arrived very early. Someone brings the child's father [. . .]. Asks how much fluid there is compared to what was in utero. I say, 'I have to look at the pictures and it will be clear'. (Participant observation diary, maternity hospital, January 2020)

Medical documents about a child's condition can not only appear before his birth, like the conclusion from the medical genetic centre in the fragment above, but sometimes they 'continue to live their own lives' even after a child is discharged from the medical institution. Most often, this happens to compile reports on the operation of the service, solve statistical problems or due to some errors in documentation:

> [The nurse dispatcher] talks about the documentation for the baby dated September 19, 2019, and says there are different names on the medical policy and the medical card. Well, apparently, last names differ. She adds the medical policy was issued to 'mummy', but the name was mixed up and there was a discrepancy. 'Some of you got their names mixed up'. And the child's daddy is from India! (Participant observation diary, Children's hospital, January 2020)

The fragment above shows that a 'paper patient' is also an 'extended patient' (for more details on this term see chapter 4), because medical documentation for a newborn includes a large amount of data on his or her parents (primarily, the mother) and, in some cases, is compiled on the basis of their documents. Officially, up to 28 days of life, a child can 'use' the insurance policy and personal insurance policy number of a parent.

The strictness of filling in various forms and documents is largely predetermined by possible sanctions from management at various levels, insurance companies, controlling state bodies and even law enforcement in some cases. This is discussed in more detail in the following sections of the chapter. Here, it is worth noting exactly how all this documentation is generated. What is included in the child's bureaucratic entity is a matter of complex negotiations between different specialists (in fact, these documents are the embodiment of this negotiated order; we use this term referring to Strauss et al. 1963) and different organisations, for each and every one of which different local formal and informal rules are relevant, in addition to the general official regulatory framework. As a result, sometimes not all components of a 'paper patient' are consistent with each other because different legal rationalities may operate at different stages and in different organisations, so sometimes there may be a direct conflict of interest. The most acute conflict of interest arises between different professional groups, such as obstetricians-gynaecologists and neonatologists:

> [Speech by the chief freelance specialist at the conference] The data (cardiocotography, Apgar scores), which obstetricians-gynaecologists provide and we look at when analysing infant mortality do not correspond to reality. 'I urge you to watch and control that carefully'. (Participant observation diary, Professional conference, November 2023)

In particular, this conflict of interest is predetermined by the differences in key performance indicators for maternity and neonatal care:

> Speaking of stats, the obstetricians did 'a great job' indicating in the children's medical card gestation period of 22 weeks and 3 days, although their mother

> hadn't got any checkup during her pregnancy. Even I resented it, as we would anyway have treated these children the best way possible, but now these parameters, which OBs have assigned, create additional pressure on us in terms of neonatal service performance. (Participant observation diary, RAC unit, January 2024)

Such conflicts of interest, regarding what data and how exactly to display in the children's medical documents, are associated not only with differences in indicators for different profiles of care (obstetrics and neonatology) but also with criteria in assessing the work of different stages of neonatal care. Observational materials and interviews include some stories about the tendency of maternity hospital employees to falsify certain medical indicators of newborns:

> At some point, a maternity hospital doctor, turning away from the RAC team members, mutely shows her nurse 'be quiet', but I did not understand what they were discussing [. . .] [already on the way to the paediatric hospital] I asked [another RAC doctor] about what maternity hospital doctors could hide (about the 'keep quiet' sign that the neonatologist showed to the nurse). Maria replied that most likely the saturation indicators had been worse even before, and not just when the RAC team arrived. It means that the maternity hospital employees don't want to take responsibility for the complication. (Participant observation diary, maternity hospital and RAC, June 2023)

> During the conversation with the RAC doctor, we switched to another topic about obstetricians-gynaecologists and neonatologists in maternity hospitals, who 'all lie', i.e. they write wrong information in medical histories. Marina always writes what she sees, and emphasise the inconsistencies between her and maternity hospitals' cards. (Participant observation diary, RAC unit, July 2023)

> I [the RAC doctor] am telling her that breathing on the right is weakened, and on the left it is crepitating, she nods and types this into the medical card. We are waiting for the test results to come out. I ask her whether they've registered the infection diagnosed or not. She says no, the discharge epicrisis will not include infection. But in my chart, I write infection as the main diagnosis, although this does not actually matter [for the routing of this patient]. (Participant observation diary, maternity hospital, January 2020)

A certain pedantry and strategy of 'not multiplying entities' in the issue of processing all documents for a child is a tangible difference between the staff of the RAC unit and other sectors of neonatal care (maternity hospitals and paediatric hospitals). This becomes especially clear when completing the 'paper body' is associated with additional difficulties, for example, a lack of official documents, language barriers between medical staff and the parents of a newborn, and (night) time for registration of patients. Below is a quote from a field diary that describes the complexities of creating appropriate and accurate documentation, as well as the differences in how medical staff working in different sectors of neonatal care approach it:

> We come in the intensive care unit of the maternity hospital, and the local doctor introduces the patient: 'Kulbe without a policy' (she says it twice with a weird accent, but I don't take it in [what is more important either] 'without a policy' or 'Kulbe') [. . .]. Alina (an RAC doctor) is trying to read the last name on the tag, swearing because it's difficult to read (the last name is 'Dzhumaninova', but it has different letters 'E' and 'I', written in other documents and on the tag). Then one more local doctor comes in with the words, 'Howdy-doody! What's kickin', chicken?!' He loudly and laughingly informs about the child, 'Easy-peasy-pumpkin-peasy!' The nickname is 'Jumanji!' He replies to Alina's indignation about an error in the last name, 'Now mommy will come, you'll ask her yourself in her native language!'
>
> Alina swears and asks local doctors to correct the tag and find out, which letter is correct (E or I), because, 'This is the only document the child has!' [. . .]
>
> Another local doctor comes in and also comments Alina's indignation about the documents, 'Well, just a second! She's got no insurance policy, no passport, nothing!' Then she continues with obscenities (but obviously good-naturedly), 'Just look at the time, this fucknut came – at 4 a.m., she can't say 'nin' or 'nen!' [. . .] Alina asks Ksenia (a nurse) if she needs help [preparing the child for transportation]. Ksenia replies 'no' and offers Alina to continue filling in the documents' [as she doesn't want to deal with docs].
>
> Alina continues to fill in the documents and shows Ksenia and me a paper that says, 'the date is indicated incorrectly' instead of the correct age or date of birth of the mother. They laugh, she comments to me 'You see this is also part of our work!' [. . .] We stop by to the intensive care unit [of a paediatric hospital], Alina hands over the baby with documents and notes that the patient is foreign. She lists vital signs, 'A Kyrgyz passport with a translation', then she corrects herself, 'Erm, an Uzbek passport with a translation'. The local doctor replies, 'I don't care'. (participant observation diary, maternity hospital, July 2023)

In at least, a few pieces of empirical evidence cited above, it can also be seen that the 'paper body' is a result of negotiation between different health professionals, which embodies the 'negotiation order' (Strauss et al. 1963) of the professionals and institutions being studied. Besides, however, they show that the bureaucratic and clinical entities of a newborn do not always completely coincide with each other. The information provided in the documents does not necessarily reflect the actual medical procedures and medication prescribed. In some cases, the 'paper body' is compiled for reasons of just utilitarian convenience: 'today I have treated twins of 470 gr. each. Both of the same weight, so one had 5 g assigned with [in the medical card] to differentiate them [in documentation]' (participant observation diary, RAC unit, January 2024). In some other instances, such a discrepancy arises just to formally justify, for example, the transfer of a child to a paediatric hospital:

> Arthur [RAC neonatologist] and Olga [neonatologist of maternity hospital] are sitting at the doctor's table. It was funny to watch Olga beginning to move her lips, when Arthur sat down at the table. She was dictating something to herself, as if she involuntarily perceived him as an observer and controller. She consulted with him on what to write in the diagnosis. 'It looks sort of sad, not enough for a [complete] diagnose here'. Apparently, she needed to justify on paper the transportation of the child. It's an interesting story about how reality is written out on paper. What will be sufficient for transportation then? (Participant observation diary, maternity hospital, January 2020)

Sometimes, on the contrary, medications (especially opiate-based painkillers, whose usage is more strictly regulated) are not indicated in the child's medical card. This is also due to the fact that the use of some medications for the treatment of newborns is not well-regulated at the legislative level:

> I ask Nadezhda (a maternity hospital doctor) if she took a Relanium injection? She says 'no, we took only paracetamol intravenously, but we did not record it. We can't!' I don't ask her why she says, 'we can't', because I suspect I know the answer [according to the instructions, it is allowed only for children older than 1 year. Although clinical recommendations and the Ministry of Health website mention dosages for newborns.] (Participant observation diary, maternity hospital, December 2019)

This may also be, however, due to the local characteristics of a particular facility, the operating hours on certain days (weekends, when there are fewer employees, or days of planned (de) hospitalisation, when the volume of paperwork increases), the time of day (at night), or even existing internal conflicts in the team:

> Talking about therapy, she mentions that we've run out of the fentanyl. I ask why she doesn't continue it. Karina explains there is a problem with writing off 'drugs' on weekends, since there are no commission members in place. So, I give my drug [which is from the resources of the RAC, not the maternity hospital]. (Participant observation diary, maternity hospital, December 2019)

> Biochemistry analysis. Olga (a maternity hospital doctor) said we should take it, but Arthur (RAC doctor) said it was not necessary (as he later explained to me the injection is given into a vein, and the veins could still be useful for other,

> more vital, injections. So, there is no need to spoil them too much, and he [the child] already has a lot of IVs in all his veins, but that analysis is sort of a formality). She objected, 'What am I supposed to tell the head of the unit?' Arthur said, 'Make a note we had arrived earlier and you didn't have time to take it'. She agreed. As Arthur told me later, their new head of the unit was not a very good person, whom many didn't trust. More confident doctors, like Olga, don't defer the head's opinion too much. But the others are afraid of dressing-down from her and act 'by the letter of the rule', sticking with the rules, so that the head of the unit doesn't become indignant. But this, in general, is counterintuitive. (Participant observation diary, maternity hospital, January 2020)

It can also be seen in most of the above fragments of empirical data that bureaucratic rules may, firstly, set some prescriptions for the newborn that are not clinically necessary for him, and following them could potentially even cause additional harm (e.g., 'spoil the veins'). Secondly, the bureaucratic nature of medical work sometimes becomes a real barrier to the provision of necessary medical care, limiting medical professionals in the speed of work, routing options, or even certain clinical assignments:

> Andreev the driver. Arthur and the members of the team (RAC) tell him to go, but the driver says he will first wait for the 'trip ticket'. The waybill is issued by the driver when starting work. 'They'll do it later', Arthur says something like this, but the driver prefers to wait for this very ticket [. . .]. Apparently, these are some shift handover formalities. (Participant observation diary, RAC unit, January 2020)

> [. . .] a few minutes later Dr. Lilieva arrived. She looked exhausted, although it was only the beginning of her shift. 'I didn't think you'd arrive so quickly!' she said. I began to ask her about the child, but she said that she hadn't really delved into [his condition], since she'd been busy with 'discharge' [completing documents necessary for dehospitalisation of patients], and there had been no time to delve into intensive care children. (Participant observation diary, maternity hospital, October 2020)

> I agreed [with a doctor of the perinatal centre, whose institution is not formally included in the RAC regional routing] that I'd examine the second child, and if he could be transferred from high frequency artificial lung ventilation apparatus to the traditional device, then I'd take him. She asked if I would be doing paperwork for my first child (official examination). I asked the doctor of the perinatal centre what was more convenient for her and whether she would follow my recommendations without my written confirmation or I should do that? She said she had no right to change antibiotics without a clinical pharmacolheadogist, so she'd better have my record to change therapy. (Participant observation diary, perinatal centre, March 2021)

New rules for prescribing certain orders and filling in the corresponding papers arise constantly. Their initiators can be legislators, control and supervisory authorities, heads of clinics or specific departments of organisations. In some cases, this is justified by the need to legally protect medical professionals, but in practice, the task of meeting formal requirements makes their work more difficult, since it requires additional time to fill in paperwork and coordinate with colleagues:

> The outgoing shift of doctors Alina and Alexander informed me there'd been announced changes at the conference. They were about the preparation of medical documentation, 'Now we need to get signatures of a few specialists for fentanyl, Relanium and Curosurf' [. . .]. I approached one of the heads of the intensive care unit, and asked about the off-label. It turned out that this was not the hospital's initiative. I was very surprised. I asked how it worked for them? He said that they filled this in for almost all children: 'This is bureaucracy, we have been living like this for a long time'. I went down to Vasily [RAC colleague] and asked, whose initiative it was, explaining again that this would greatly complicate our work, because we would have to fill in additional paper for each child and find someone to sign it. (Participant observation diary, children's hospital, November 2019)

In a sense, medical organisations are not only a place of clinical observation and treatment of a child, but also a place of 'birth and treatment' of his or her documents ('paper body'), that is, official and social statuses, which, among other things, allow compensation for payment for medical services provided:

> Sometimes you get a medical history after discharge, but you can't issue an invoice, because the package of documents that the child had when entering, accordingly, hasn't changed until his discharge. You cannot put it into the payment system, because hospitalised depends on how much assistance we provide. If this is mandatory health insurance, then there is a big difference between the medical policy of our city or the policy of another territory. If these are high technology services [and corresponding funding], they are generally only available to citizens of the Russian Federation, who have permanent registration in our city. Therefore, 3 people, I mean 3 nurses, (nurses, because these are people with medical knowledge and experience in our organisation, who know who a patient is, where he's from, with what prognosis for treatment he arrived and what will be required to do further) check all patients admitted to our 24/7 inpatient beds. Everyone, who is admitted, has their diagnoses checked. Then, depending on whether a patient is a Russian citizen or not, resident of the city or not, [a certain decision is made]. Next, they contact the parents and work, in parallel, with the clinicians, so that the entire missing package of documents

is completed during the child's treatment in the hospital. (An interview with a deputy chief physician for administrative and expert work, October 2023)

The above quote clearly shows that the need to create a complete (and 'correct') 'paper body' of a newborn arises largely due to the fact that the institution, which medical care was provided in, is obliged to find the way to reimburse the material resources spent on it. However, funds for the provision of neonatal care and its material support are not the only resources necessary for the operation of the service. The following subsection details what types of resources are attracted by neonatologists and nurses and how they are distributed across different sectors and different institutions.

Resources, Their Distribution and Shortage

Material Resources

In many sociocultural contexts and different cases, even within institutionalised obstetric care, the birth of a child is viewed as a relatively 'natural' event that does not require specialised expertise, technical devices and medications (Borozdina 2018; Avdeeva 2020; Temkina et al. 2022). The field under study is empirically isolated from this debate on the conventional boundaries of 'technocratic' and 'holistic' approaches to maternity and neonatal care (Davis-Floyd 2001), since this applies entirely to cases requiring resuscitation, intensive care, or hospitalisation in specialised hospitals. Thus, not only professionally and organisationally, but also materially, the environment of the empirical field under study differs from less medicalised and less technologised contexts of newborn care. Technical and medical support for the work of neonatologists and nurses in certain situations turns out to be no less important component of care than their professional knowledge and skills. This paragraph shows exactly what kind of material resources and infrastructure of the neonatal service are involved in the treatment of the physical body of a newborn, as well as in his or her 'paper body'.

Various medications are a very important component of the material support for the work of neonatologists and nurses. As has already been shown in the previous paragraph, the use of some of them is strictly regulated by legislation, clinical recommendations, local protocols of medical organisations, as well as informal rules. The possibility of using a particular drug depends on a combination of professional logic (primarily the assessment of the most optimal clinical outcomes), legal regulation and its accessibility (both financial and physical):

> [from the speech of the chief freelance neonatologist at the conference] 'Please, pay attention to the following fact – the most effective regimen was developed by Japanese doctors. The pain relief regimen is fentanyl 1–2 mcg/kg/hour + midazolam 0.05–0.2 mg/kg /hour, within 72 hours. This may be difficult to provide, but there was no fentanyl in maternity hospitals before either [before the opening of neonatal intensive care units in maternity hospitals]'. (Participant observation diary, professional conference, November 2023)

As was already shown in the first chapter, professional expertise and initiatives often 'win' in the competition between bureaucratic rules, economic rationality and professionalism. Therefore, it becomes possible to introduce the most effective techniques into the practice of doctors. The above quote from the diary shows there are quite successful examples of the introduction of a particular drug into practice, even though it also confirms the fact that it is unevenly available across different institutions and different sectors of neonatal care. The absence of any device or medication in the maternity hospital can be interpreted by its staff as a symbolic isolation of this sector of neonatal care, which is focused primarily on 'healthy children':

> On the way to the post, I ask the nurse of the maternity hospital if they have perfolgan or paracetamol [different trade names for the drug acetaminophen]. She looks at me with amazed eyes and graciously says (in a kind way with a smile), 'Arthur, what are you talking about!? We have never had such medicines and, after all, we are a maternity hospital, so we must assist with birth to healthy children and discharge them home'. I ask my [RAC] nurse to go to the ambulance for 'perfolgan'. (Participant observation diary, maternity hospital, December 2019)

In some cases, however, the lack of necessary medications really affects the well-being and condition of a newborn patient:

> We've run out of fentanyl and I ask the doctor (of the maternity hospital): 'Do you have any fentanyl?' She says they don't. I say we've run out and nothing's at hand, since we carry only one ampoule [per trip]. She says, sort of absently, either to me or to herself, 'Yes, it [the sedation effect] will end now . . . and the child will wake up!' (Participant observation diary, maternity hospital, January 2020)

Such exhaustible 'resources' can be not necessarily expensive or paperwork-exhausting drugs, but also, for example, nutrition for newborns. The difficulty of providing the necessary nutrition for patients (including rising prices) may lead to attempts to change the overall approach to the hospitalisation of newborns, to the breastfeeding promotion, and even to the creation of an entire logistics infrastructure:

> [A chief specialist speaks at a conference for neonatologists], 'Recently there was a meeting of the formulary commission at our children's hospital. They reported that the pricing policy for everything had changed. The consumption of the sterile mixture had increased, and its cost had increased by 2.5 times. However, necrotising enterocolitis persists. This is our work with you, we need to organise it so that at the stages of the neonatal care involve a mother. Breastfeeding is not only economically beneficial [but also better for health reasons]. It will require elaborating logistics to consider mothers, when their children are hospitalised'. (Participant observation diary, professional conference, November 2023)

Important material resources for the neonatology service are not only the medications themselves but also devices that help measure them and ensure their infusion. Just like medications, the number of syringe dispensers (or infusion pumps) may be limited and unevenly distributed both between institutions and different patients. In some severe cases, they can be 'borrowed' from the maternity hospital where the baby is hospitalised:

> Arthur [RAC doctor] and his team are counting infusion pumps. There are only four available [with the RAC team], but the patient needs six. It means you either have to rearrange something – turn something off, or borrow from the hospital. Employees of the maternity hospital firstly say, 'We can't give anything, everything is reserved'. But then continue: 'Erm, you'll come back, though. Alright, take as many as you need!' (Participant observation diary, maternity hospital, January 2020)

It is interesting to note that the number of infusion pumps required for each particular patient is a material embodiment of the severity of his or her condition; that is, the more critical the child's condition is, the more drugs are required to be administered simultaneously, and subsequently the more infusion pumps are to be connected:

> Ksenia (an RAC nurse) asks: 'How many infusion pumps do we need?' Alina (an RAC doctor) answers, 'I hope one is enough'. (I note to myself that the number of infusion pumps is a kind of local scale of the severity of the patient's condition) [. . .]. [Later on the same day, but in a different maternity hospital] while we are getting out of the car, Alina says to Ksenia, 'I hope for 5 infusion pumps!' Ksenia replies, 'Are you kidding?!' (I understand that the child, weighing 600 g, requires more complex therapy). (Participant observation diary, RAC unit, July 2023)

Infusion pumps, mobile incubators with heat and moisture regulation, artificial lung ventilation apparatuses (which can also differ in the degree of technological performance and effectiveness), consumables and components for them, ambulances and many other technical devices make up the complex infrastructure of neonatological care. The distribution of these resources crosses departmental and institutional boundaries, and the lack of such resources for one patient can lead to changes in the treatment of another one:

> I'm going to find out if there are available reducers for oxide. There is none of them in the corridors of the intensive care unit. I go back to the therapist [the employee in charge of medical equipment] and say that I didn't find anything. He replies, 'That means we've got no one!' The head of the intensive care unit, Dr. Petrov, is at the same post. I tell him that I am going to see a child with severe complications and ask if they can remove the oxide from any child [treated in the NICU]. He points to the child at the same post and says that the patient is no longer very dependent on oxide, and the head of the unit is trying to take him away from it. 'We may give it a go', he says. He begins to cut off the oxide. I'm going to get some wrenches and disconnect the reducer from the cylinder. I come back 5–10 minutes later, the child has good saturation, I call Petrov and ask him if I may remove the reducer? He allows it. I remove the reducer, and we go. (Participant observation diary, children's hospital, March 2020)

Not all parts of this complex infrastructure are 'exhaustible resources' or ones exchangeable between different organisations and units, as described above. Some elements of the material environment may seem completely external to a newborn patient and the work of the neonatologists. Nevertheless, based on interviews and observational data, it is clear that the infrastructure of neonatal care often extends beyond the confines of an ambulance car or a specific health care facility and can involve the urban environment and even the cross-regional transport system.

Infrastructure of Institutions, City and Country

Previous researches suggest that infrastructure and the material environment can have a direct and formative impact on social life, including the health care system (Edwards 2002; Mokhov & Novkunskaya 2021). The interaction of social actors and non-human actors in the process of creating, using and changing infrastructures is the subject of interest of the whole theoretical and epistemological approach – 'Science and technology studies' (see, for example, Hughes 1993; Star 1999; Mol 2002). This paragraph does not go into the details of the theoretical discussion about the impact of technologies and material infrastructures on the professional practices of doctors and nurses and the patient's condition but tries to empirically outline how different elements of the material environment can participate in the provision of care to the very small body of a newborn patient (the smallest patient, who was transported by the staff of the resuscitation and advisory team during the fieldwork, weighed 380g).

Although transporting a resuscitated newborn is the daily work of the resuscitation and advisory service and a fairly probable event for maternity hospitals (especially large institutions, where several thousand children are born a year), many institutions remain technically unprepared for such situations, and even the installation of a convenient ramp for a heavy neonatal transport incubator can remain a big problem (which sometimes is not solved for years):

> Since Tatyana Yuryevna (main specialist of the region) is usually busy, and she has many problems to solve, I take this opportunity to ask her to resolve the issue with the ramp in the X-maternity hospital. She listens to me and writes it down, promising to try to figure it out. But usually this results in nothing. This is not our first time asking her. (Participant observation diary, children's hospital, January 2020)

> We are discussing with the driver how poorly organised the access points for transporting newborns are (there are holes everywhere, inconvenient entrances and ramps). He is telling me once he was testing a new ramp in the X-maternity hospital on the RAC car and had to either accept it or not. (We visited that maternity hospital earlier on that day.) He says, at first it was built narrow and short (not suitable for the ambulance and unloading the incubator, so Alexander [the driver] did not approve it). The ramp was redone later. (Participant observation diary, maternity hospital, July 2023)

A convenient ramp in a medical institution is an understandable and expected part of the neonatal care infrastructure. This and other infrastructure that make up the external material environment, such as convenient access to entrances and city roads, most often are not considered necessary components of the path of a newborn in the event of his or her medical routing. However, they turn into physically tangible obstacles that affect both the travel time and its 'smoothness':

> We don't have far to go, but now as we have a baby in the car, I notice how many potholes and speed bumps there are on the roads. The ambulance driver is trying to pass them very-very carefully, but it is still sensitive. There are cars parked in several places on the hospital grounds, blocking our car's access. The driver turns on the signals and is indignant at why they are there. (Participant observation diary, RAC unit, June 2023)

The children's hospital, where most of the ethnographic observations were carried out, officially has the status of a city hospital. However, the complexity and quality of medical care provided here make this institution 'attractive' for residents of other regions. Thus, in some cases, the patient's hospitalisation infrastructure ends up stretching over thousands of kilometres and hours of travel:

> [In the city hospital there are] children from other regions, who either end up in an emergency ambulance, when they visit our beautiful city and get sick here, or targeted children, who come to us to receive medical care on referrals from other regions. You see, it is surprising to me that children from Sakhalin, Kamchatka, the Urals, and Khabarovsk are trying to come to us. And when I ask the question, 'You can't get treatment closer [to your native town], can you?', they say, 'No, we can't. It's easier for us to be going by train for a week and by air for 14 hours, but get treatment at your hospital'. (An interview with the deputy chief physician for administrative and expert work, October 2023)

Infrastructure Repairs

As mentioned earlier, many infrastructures associated in Russia with key life cycle events (including birth) are characterised by multiple breakdowns and gaps and therefore require constant adjustment and repair (Mokhov & Novkunskaya 2021). Neonatal intensive care is no exception. On the one hand, it includes many high-tech devices, as described above, but on the other hand, it experiences a constant shortage of various resources and requires 'manual' adjustment, repair and even the invention of 'vernacular instruments':

> I return to my conversation with Arthur. He shows the reducer and reminds how to install it. Afterwards he clarifies that the regulator does not work either, but quickly explains, 'take the system from the dropper, cut it off, insert it in here, and adjust it, using the wheel'. (Participant observation diary, RAC unit, December 2019)

> [an RAC nurse upon coming back] disinfects the medical gloves, filled with water. They were in the neonatal transport incubator. I ask why do they needed them at all? For cooling? She replies, [they are used] to press, compact the mattress (sort of shock absorption) so that it doesn't shake so much, especially for lightweight children. (Participant observation diary, RAC unit, July 2023)

> At some point, an incredible discussion of equipment begins. Arthur says that he soldered some wiring. He is showing it to Maria, but it turns out that some transitional part seems to be missing, which apparently, as they assume, is lying around somewhere 'in the bag'. Maria says she took some part from the washing machine from home for the contours, seemingly to better hold and secure them. Something like that. Also, she has some similar parts in the plastic bag, they may be suitable for attaching contours, too (for the artificial lung ventilation apparatus). I am amazed in my heart. Moreover, all this is intended for a

high-tech Swiss-made incubator, as far as I get it. (Participant observation diary, RAC unit, January 2020)

Constant repair of infrastructure, on the one hand, is a kind of customisation, that is, the optimisation of devices and consumables for specific work features. On the other hand, it is caused by a lack of material resources, both the equipment itself and the funds to repair it if it breaks down. This is due not only to the cost of high-tech equipment but also to a number of bureaucratic and even political features of Russian healthcare. One of them is a complex and lengthy process of state procurement of any equipment or medicine. This procedure requires holding a tender, drawing up tender documentation in a certain way (so that the supply corresponds to medical effectiveness and not just economic efficiency), but most importantly, it takes up a lot of time:

> Alina (an RAC doctor) asks the maternity hospital staff at the entrance to call the elevator, but we are standing in front of the elevator for two minutes (because the service lift, which the transport incubator fits into, cannot be called just by a button). Ksenia (an RAC nurse) says jokingly, 'It's the age of high technology, and we are waiting for the elevator! By the way, when are they going to give out tablets?' [to replace paperwork] Alina replies it won't happen until the new year. (Participant observation diary, maternity hospital, July 2023)

The imperfection of material infrastructures constantly requires the inclusion of people in their work. This happens not only while the 'fixing' of certain devices but also routinely, when a person 'by design' is part of the operation of some device (such as the lift with a lift attendant), but it also happens spontaneously, when the involvement of outsiders allows medical staff to save their own efforts and time:

> We enter the territory of the X-maternity hospital, and Alina warns us that now they are going to pull out the incubator, which weighs 300 kg, but 'the ramp is still a sorry story'. She asks if I have pins or if I'm pregnant, because . . . then I can help. But it turns out that there is a second RAC car parked at the same maternity hospital, and Alina joyfully says, 'Great! We have Tolya, Tolya will help!' (talking about the driver of the second team of the RAC). (Participant observation diary, RAC unit, July 2023)

> In the lift, Arthur reduces the child's oxygen from 35 to 30 per cent and at some point, jokes about saving oxygen. He says the more independence a child has, when breathing, the better. There is also some other rationality, though, i.e. if you save oxygen and the cylinder doesn't run out, you won't have to change it yourself. These are resources, too, although not material (oxygen is not expensive), but physical and time-related. The next team will change the cylinder. (Participant observation diary, RAC unit, January 2020)

Thus, medical professionals providing care for newborns can be conceptualised as a social resource, which is also unevenly distributed and may 'run out':

> I complain to her that when I arrived [at the maternity hospital], I saw an abandoned doctor [she was caring for a seriously sick child by herself]. Anna (the head of the maternity department) puts on a serious face and seems to be thinking. Then she begins to explain that the second doctor left for classes in the morning, the nurses at this time have a lot of their own work, which they cannot help but do, and . . . in general Maria (the only doctor left) is sort of unhappy and always 'attracts troubles'. Then I ask her if the city [authorities] bought them the 'Fabian' [an expert-level ventilator]. She says she doesn't know; she is tired of asking them for something, so they [the maternity hospital] have nothing [equipment] to work with, and they don't buy anything. The only thing, she is waiting for, is just two tables for the maternity ward . . . [paid for] by the deputies. (Participant observation diary, maternity hospital, January 2020)

The workload on medical professionals and, subsequently, the timeliness and quality of care that they can provide to newborns are directly dependent on a number of conditions and resources, such as financing, material support, operating hours of the institution and management decisions. This is how this interdependence is described in the following situation, which continues the story of waiting for a service elevator in a maternity hospital:

> There is still no lift operator, no one answers calls from the reception staff. Ksenia (an RAC nurse) begins to dial the number, indicated on the lift. I hear the phone ringing (somewhere on the first floor), but no one picks up. Alina (an RAC doctor) says that she will go up to the 3rd floor [the one where NICU is] and try to find someone. She leaves on the passenger lift, and suddenly at this time a service lift with the operator arrives. On the one hand, she [the operator] sort of apologises and explains, 'I went out for dinner, and everyone is quitting, so I had my tongue engaged with the barmaid, gabbing away. Today's her last day of work!' On the other hand, she seems to be complaining and absolving herself of responsibility for her absence, 'With the new hospital administration, everyone is leaving, we have 50% of the employees left, but salaries are still being cut' [. . .]
>
> On the 3rd floor, we are met by Alina and a young local neonatologist. They both ask what the problem was in calling the lift operator. Ksenia replies, 'dinner', but Alina sympathetically recalls, 'Oh, they're making layoffs!' The local doctor agrees, 'Well, yes, here you must be Jack of all trades. So, the lift operator, maybe, is working alone for several departments!' [. . .]
>
> The local doctor complains that their artificial lung ventilation has broken down (she mentions some brand) and even Arthur came with contours and checked

> up. 'It's expensive to repair, it's expensive to call someone from Moscow [to repair]!' Alina jokes, 'You have a very economical new chief doctor!' The local doctor replies, 'Right, soon he'll be delivering lunch himself!' (Participant observation diary, maternity hospital, July 2023)

The above quote shows that a reduction in staff and an increase in the load on remaining employees are caused not only by a person's dependence on the inevitable participation in the work of infrastructure, but also by the difficulty of converting different resources within one institution, that is, restrictions on maternity hospital financing and certain management decisions. In turn, the lack of human resources leads to malfunctioning of technical devices and additional time costs, which turn out to be most critical for cases requiring emergency care. Time appears to be another key resource of the field under study, since, firstly, it is critically important in the most emergency situations, and, secondly, it becomes an additional dimension of trading between different medical professionals and institutions.

Time as a Resource

> Alina does not want to rush to leave [the RAC unit], since the child was born at 1 p.m., and he needs to be administered with a second Curosurf [a surfactant drug to improve lung function], this is a maternity hospital drug (the RAC doesn't have it), and the maternity hospital is most likely to save money and leave it all 'to chance' (without the second injection). Alina and Ksenia discuss that they do not understand what the maternity hospital's staff is counting on, because . . . no any RAC doctor will transport the child without the second injection.
>
> They go on, saying that the X-maternity hospital is the one, which children must be taken out from, as quickly as possible, because . . . there is a large flow of patients and they cannot take adequate care of difficult children. They also discuss that there is still difficulty in 'transferring' a child to the intensive care unit in a children's hospital, for example, at night, since 'no one wants to work at night'. But sometimes it happens that by the morning someone gets worse, another child, requiring help, is born, and as a result four patients for intensive care units accumulate at once. (Participant observation diary, RAC unit, July 2023)

In the observation diary excerpted above, time emerges as a significant resource in several dimensions of neonatal care. Firstly, the 'wait' strategy, even when calling for clinically complex cases, happens to be an opportunity to save the time of the visiting team at the expense of the resources (use of the drug) of the maternity hospital. Secondly, the lack of time to provide care to difficult patients in some institutions is an important factor for determining the priority of resuscitation team visits and for scheduling the entire service, too. Thirdly, the time of day (night) is defined as another condition that affects the success of routing, in particular, the readiness of the receiving institution to register the child. Finally, untimely departures and transportation of patients can lead to a 'cumulative effect', which will be much more difficult to cope with, again due to a lack of material and human resources.

In this sense, the resuscitation and advisory service also turns into a tool for redistributing time and labour resources between different sectors of neonatal care. This position of doctors and nurses of RAC teams predetermines the communicative and even emotional register, which they will be met in by employees of maternity hospitals and paediatric hospitals:

> In the hallway of the emergency room, I turned to the woman behind the glass desk and asked if she knew about the child's transfer to the children's hospital, and explained that they were waiting for us in the intensive care unit. To this, she rather rudely told me, 'Why are you addressing me?' and waved towards another woman sitting at a specially equipped table in the corridor of the reception room, adding, 'You should go there!' (I believe she thought that we'd brought a child, because this was a common story with queues in the emergency room waiting for boxing). I approached another woman, who looked more friendly, and explained the situation that we were from a children's hospital and would probably pick up a child from their NICU, that they were waiting for us, and asked how we could get there. She listened to me and said she'd call the intensive care unit and find out everything. [The dissatisfaction of employees is very clearly evident in the reception areas of all maternity hospitals. They sigh with relief, when they realise that we have not brought a woman, but are going to take away a child. Maternity hospital doctors, when giving us children, are always happy to see us, even at night. Children's hospital doctors and nurses often grumble, when we bring children (especially when they have a lot of work to do or at night)]. (Participant observation diary, maternity hospital, January 2020)

Distribution of the load between different institutions and specialists is also carried out within one sector. As a rule, trips of different RAC teams are carried out in a certain order, taking into account both the (assumed) complexity of the case and the overall workload on a particular doctor:

> A consultant doctor said that there was a child with positive COVID in the X-maternity hospital (working as a COVID hospital) and he needed to be transferred to the X-infectious diseases hospital. She said she didn't know, whom to send, 'You see if I send you now, then they'll ask me why I sent a machine with an oscillator for such a child'. I told her that during my previous duty, Dr. Kruglova transferred a child with COVID, and she was already tired of those personal protective equipment changes. In addition, the Head of medicine

> [Deputy Chief Physician for Medical Affairs or Medical Work] was interested in who'd transferred that child, since she said that the same doctors and nurses should not go for such children (this is due to additional payments so that they are distributed evenly among all staff). (Participant observation diary, RAC unit, October 2020)

The above quote from the diary shows that the distribution of financial resources and remuneration is also taken into account when the workload is distributed among different employees. The next paragraph of this section describes this dimension of the work of the neonatology services in a little more detail.

Hospital Losses

This paragraph is devoted to the financial system of the service under study. It is in this dimension that a newborn patient most often appears as 'a unit of account', since the medical organisation requests reimbursement for the resources spent on his or her treatment and transportation, based on the diagnosis and medical history. The nuances of financing medical care may be completely invisible to the child's family, since in most cases, citizens of the Russian Federation do not pay for medical care directly, but pay monthly taxes to the health insurance fund. The absence of direct payments to medical organisations creates an image of 'free healthcare' among patients and their relatives. However, financial flows within the medical care system are more like its blood flow, which is not always visible but which is critical for ensuring its vital functions.

Payments for medical care provided can become noticeable (and even very sensitive) for patients and their relatives only if a patient and his or her parents do not have Russian citizenship (this is discussed in more detail in the final section of the chapter), or if they initially applied to private medical organisations (maternity hospitals), or if they want to pay for some additional commercial services. However, for administrators and managers of medical organisations, no any healthcare provided is free. The only question is who exactly should make up for the costs. An important job in this regard is the correct execution of financial documents and invoices that are issued either to the territorial mandatory health insurance fund, or to the city budget, or to some federal sources (e.g., when paying for high-tech care). If the financial costs of medical care were not reimbursed to the medical organisation, then they are defined in the categories of 'losses', since the medical institution is forced to pay for them from its own budget. Here is how the deputy chief physician, whose main professional task is to correctly prepare financial documentation, says about that:

> Well, little by little, somehow, you begin to realise where, what, and how it would be possible to organise the work of doctors and recording of the medical documents properly, so that the losses of our hospital. . . . So that they are reduced. Just imagine, when I was appointed the head of the accounting department, our hospital's losses were 13% of the invoices issued. We've boiled this down to 0.2% of invoices. I mean when this began, it's scary to say, 18 years ago, our financial plan for MHI fund alone was 600 million. And I was horrified, because, by and large, our department, which I headed, was responsible for every penny of the invoice, making sure that everything was invoiced correctly, according to the law, and insurance companies could not fine us for any lack of a comma or signatures in the medical cards. When the financial plan came over more than a billion, I just was no longer afraid. Now our financial plan is 2 billion 200 million a year. This is a bare to MHI fund. Plus, we have commercial and high technology services [. . .]. I mean, among other things, our hospital provides high-tech medical care, according to quotas of the federal Ministry of Health. Besides, there is HTMC in compulsory medical insurance, it's another type, but also a certain source of funding. We have agreements with neighbouring regions to provide targeted high-tech types of medical care for children and residents of their regions. This is also a whole package of approvals. Also, there is voluntary medical insurance, cash in the pay desk. In general, there are a lot of things in here. (An interview with the deputy chief physician for administrative and expert work, October 2023)

A long quote from the interview is provided specifically to illustrate how many different sources of funding (and therefore different financial documents) have to be taken into account in the work of medical organisations, providing neonatal care. This story also contains a description of the fact that in recent years, the financial plan of the institution has only been growing, while the hospital's 'losses', on the contrary, have been reduced. A key condition for such economic success is the painstaking completion of documents (down to the comma), which reduces the likelihood of fines from insurance companies. However, avoiding fines is not the only way to improve the funding of a service. According to another informant (the head of the neonatal department of the maternity hospital), compiling the patient's 'paper body' in a certain way in some cases allows to increase reimbursement of the medical care provided to him or her:

> I say [to the management of the maternity hospital], 'Listen, are you sane?' I say, 'look, a child was admitted, you opened his medical history, put in high-tech medical care, closed the medical history, opened it [a new history] according to compulsory medical insurance, back and forth . . '. And they are like, 'You mean it was possible, wasn't it?' I say, 'You bet!' They are like, 'Well, sort of like, no, we can't do that'. Then they called for lawyers, the lawyers mulled it over. We had five-six meetings later there, that kind of

> thing. . . . They eventually came to the conclusion that it was really possible! And in fact, it turns out [. . .] the story is like this. I mean when he [a child] came from the delivery room, he had no medical card. He had a neonatal record. You give him an injection of surfactants, register it as respiratory distress syndrome, and close it [the first medical history] and then you open another history of a NICU patient. After ten days you transfer him to the second stage, close the previous history and open a new one on prematurity. Here he will be lying as if born prematurely, until he's been discharged home. You have already earned money there. . . . You know the quotas there are large, 450–500 thousand [rubles]. So, in fact, you've just earned a ton of money. (An interview with the head of the neonatal department of the maternity hospital, May 2023)

It is the field of neonatal care that turns out to be the most 'intensive' in terms of funding opportunities, even compared to other areas of paediatrics. This is due both to the high symbolic status of a newborn in the pronatalist agenda of the state (see the next section of the chapter on this issue) and to the fact that resuscitation and hospitalisation of newborns is considered to be more high-tech care with higher tariffs. One of the informants even describes the logic of the economic mode of this service provision in terms of a 'capitalist conveyor belt':

> *R.:* Well, it's like a capitalist conveyor belt, yes, something like that, the one for making money.
>
> *I.:* Neonatology, in particular?
>
> *R.:* Yes. That's all because there is a patient, he has a disease, these diseases are treated, using high-tech medical care, well, and there are a lot of documents for the child to be filled in and closed. That means a lot of paperwork. That kind of thing. [. . .] It is well funded, so it is profitable to do it. If you have a lot of these patients and you treat them in large numbers, that's pretty good money for institutions. (An interview with the head of the paediatric intensive care unit, April 2023)

The nuances of compiling a patient history and financial documents remain largely in the jurisdiction of healthcare managers (heads of departments, deputy chief physicians, and other managers). However, the need to 'earn money' (to receive compensation for the assistance provided, especially high-tech, as the most highly paid) creates a kind of competition between institutions.

The previous paragraph described that patient routing between different healthcare organisations was also a means of distributing the workload among different healthcare professionals and institutions. However, if employees of maternity hospitals and paediatric hospitals are most often not happy with the additional burden in the form of a seriously ill patient in terms of effort and time spent, then in terms of the distribution of financial flows and due to the principle of per capita financing ('money follows a patient'), they are more likely to compete for a newborn:

> At children's hospital, a nurse and a doctor meet us. The doctor is worried about the child. I say the child is 'good', and he has no problems but paresis. I ask her if they are waiting for someone else. She replies, 'No, we've barely talked them into [giving us] this one, almost cajoled!' Then she asks me if there are many children in the city. I answer there are children, of course [who require hospitalisation in paediatric hospitals]. She chuckles, 'But we don't deserve it!' (apparently, they have few children, and she is unhappy with this). (Participant observation diary, children's hospital, October 2020).

The dominance of such 'market' logic (Freidson 2001) over professional one is manifested primarily in the need to 'fill beds', that is, to ensure the maximum possible load on the department within the framework of economic feasibility:

> I ask what's the matter? Why do they [the neonatal intensive care unit in the paediatric hospital] want a transfer [of the child to themselves]? I try to soften that question, and add that I am ready to go for the child right away, I don't mind going there and pick him up, but I see a certain inconsistency in the work of the NICU. 'In some cases, you ask to let them lie longer [children in the maternity hospital], then you want to transfer them within the first hours of life'. I ask him, 'What is your tactic for dealing with low weight babies?' He sighs, 'We don't have any tactics', and begins to say that there really is no incubator freely available right now, but there are six free places in the department, and therefore children must be taken. (Participant observation diary, children's hospital, December 2019)

In the maternity hospital sector, the same logic of maximising 'benefit' (i.e., maximising the amount of the bill that can be issued to the insurance company) can be seen in reverse situations, when a newborn is 'registered' (i.e., they inform of the need to transfer him to a paediatric hospital) and he or she is transferred only after the period of stay, which is necessary to comply with the tariff, has passed:

> We're going to look at the baby. The child is at the next post, his weight is 1,100 g, he's on a ventilator, stable. I ask why he is not registered. The maternity hospital doctor replies that the head of the unit told him to register the child only as the day was over, but at the same time asked him to transfer the patient today. (Participant observation diary, maternity hospital, December 2019)

In the above fragment of the diary, the time of handing over the child to the staff of the resuscitation and consultation centre turns out to be an accurate calculation between the need to properly 'close the medical history' at the maternity hospital stage and the need to hand over a complex patient on time, minimising the risks of his or her deterioration. In some cases, the desire of maternity hospital management to prolong the stay of complex patients leads to additional pressure and increased workload on those doctors, who are directly responsible for their treatment:

> The head of the maternity department and I understand that the children are extremely difficult and need to be transferred to a large hospital. Leaving the maternity hospital, I say goodbye to the head, 'It's time for you to go home and rest', because he stays late at work every day. That same evening at 8.30 p.m. he writes, 'Come!' I call him back. He is still in the hospital. He says that a child is deteriorating, and he decided to transfer him. 'They [the maternity hospital administration] don't let me go home until you arrive'. I suggest he go home straight away, 'We'll be there in 20 minutes, go home'. But he meets us at the maternity hospital without ever leaving home, although it was already 9.30 p.m. He says, 'I'm run off my feet with him, I did everything, but nothing helps!' We begin to prepare the child for transportation [. . .]. He is forced to stay with seriously ill children, whom the administration asks not to transfer too quickly and to go on treating them in the maternity hospital. (Participant observation diary, maternity hospital, March 2021)

The policy of maternity hospitals is aimed at keeping patients, whose treatment is paid at a higher rate, for as long as possible. This is not the only manifestation of market logic in the field of medical care provided to newborns. For example, within an institution, a child may be assigned to different departments if the stay in one of them (most often commercial) is paid in a different amount or from a different source:

> The maternity hospital doctor asked me to pick up one of the children. She said that he would now be brought in from his mother, and added that he was still registered in intensive care, 'he earns us money' [the child was born with meconium aspiration and needed mechanical ventilation for seven hours, but at the time of transfer there was a significant improvement and the doctors handed him over to his mother not for long]. (Participant observation diary, maternity hospital, October 2020)

Third-level maternity hospitals (perinatal centres) can also, to some extent, influence the overall flow of patients, accepting not only patients requiring specialised care. This policy corresponds to market logic, where a woman herself chooses the place of delivery, but it is not approved by the professional community and is described quite critically, primarily from the point of view of the quality of care provided to newborns and their clinical outcomes:

> *R.:* Healthy women did not give birth in our [perinatal centre in another region]. We had this story of another kind there, it wasn't like that. What does it [name of the perinatal centre of the region of study] do?
>
> I2.: Yes, they take everyone.
>
> *R.:* Yes, healthy women give birth there, they are trying to earn dough. Well, in fact, it turns out that, of course, in this case, your delivery room, you have to empty it.
>
> *I1.:* Why does giving birth to healthy women mean 'earning money'?
>
> *I2.:* Because they are paid more. . . . The more you give birth, the more you earn. And they don't just specialise in what they should [pathologies and preterm birth]. They take this piece and want to take another, larger piece. Of course, it results in, well, a very large flow, and this is already harm to those children who are born. (An interview with the head of the neonatal department of the maternity hospital, May 2023)

Emergency services staff also have some ability to influence the patient's documentation history (which in turn allows them to request greater compensation for the care provided). For example, the final tariff may depend on what technical devices were used at this stage, as well as what is considered as an indicator of the severity of the patient's condition:

> The RAC doctors report on what happened during the day, but since I'm sitting in the back, I can't really see who's talking. In general, everything is formal. As I understand it, they report on the condition and diagnoses of transferred children. The doctor in the white coat [chief] is nodding mostly. Suddenly, he asks about some child, '[Was he] wearing a mask or not?' (i.e. an oxygen mask or not. The tariff, which the call is paid at, depends on this fact). The doctor answers, doubting it for a second, 'Yes, with a mask on'. 'That's it!' the head [in the white coat] says edifyingly. (Participant observation diary, RAC unit, January 2020)

From the above fragments of empirical evidence, it might seem that the routing of newborn patients depends primarily on clinical need or bureaucratic/economic rationality and does not take into account the interests of the 'extended patient'. In most cases (in particular, when it comes to emergency care), nothing else can influence the professional decisions made. However, sometimes the transfer of a child becomes the subject of complex negotiations and trading between the maternity hospital and the receiving hospital, sort of the struggle for good performance of the service as a whole, the clinical indicators of the child himself, and the interests of the mother (or parents):

> Dr. Ivanova (an RAC doctor) asks to measure the child's blood pressure and saturation. The maternity hospital doctor doesn't want to, but after a while she brings a monitor and they measure the pressure. Dr. Ivanova explains to the mother that it is better to transfer a patient to another hospital in the interests of her child. The mother says, though, that the chief of medicine has already talked to her, and she will not go to another hospital, because there are some problems to stay with the child. Dr. Ivanova asks the mother to make an entry in the call card and confirm that she categorically refuses to be transferred to the X-hospital. (Participant observation diary, maternity hospital, April 2022)

The next day, the child was diagnosed with cardiac pathology, and he was transferred to the hospital, which his mother refused to go to. This situation demonstrates the conflict between professional and consumerist logics. On the one hand, a mother has the right to choose which hospital her child will be routed to. On the other hand, a doctor does not always have the opportunity to prove/explain to the mother that in some situations, household amenities and comfort should fade into the background, especially when it comes to possible clinical outcomes for her child. Refusal to be hospitalised in any institution or to receive medical care at all is not the only way parents can influence the trajectory of their newborn child in the neonatal care system. Depending on the available resources (both economic and social), some families can initiate quite complex transfers that do not fit into standard patient routing within the regional system of neonatal care:

> I was sitting in the office with Dr. Potapova (she worked as a RAC consultant), when at about 5 p.m. the chief of medicine called her and said that he had 'stirred up' a complicated transfer. He wanted to know if any of the doctors from the federal perinatal centre had called us at the RAC [. . .]. As it turned out, twin premature children (600 and 700 g) were born, in this perinatal centre. And their mother had another child, who'd been treated in our hospital with a severe malformation about 5–6 years ago. The child was successfully operated on, and as I took it in, the mother subsequently provided sponsorship to the hospital. This mother did not like the treatment at the perinatal centre, and she contacted our administration with a request to arrange a transfer to our hospital. (Participant observation diary, children's hospital, March 2021)

The strongest influence of parents on the routing and hospitalisation of a child is noticeable in the sector of commercial health services, when they initially try to pay for more comfortable conditions of childbirth, additional services, the possibility of a partner [a spouse] being present during labour, and the right to exercise their agency to a greater extent (Temkina and Rivkin-Fish 2020; Temkina et al. 2022). Commercial childbirth can occur both in private institutions (there are four private maternity hospitals in the city under study) and in 'commercial' departments of state-funded institutions. As a result, the latter may lay down informal rules that prioritise the provision of medical care to those patients who receive it under a commercial contract (rather than a MHI policy).

However, most often the 'contract for childbirth' is concluded between a woman and the obstetric team, and this practically does not take into account the interests of the neonatology service staff. Therefore, neonatologists of state maternity hospitals can position themselves as employees who have no commercial relations with a patient's parents and are guided exclusively by the professional logic of work:

> Dr. Lilieva (a neonatologist at the maternity hospital) told the midwife that she couldn't [conduct a checkup], because she was transferring the child, and they [doctors] had warned them the day before that it would be difficult at the weekend (apparently, there were very few doctors). Anyway, she had no time for 'paid' children. [It's about the priority of self-supporting childbirth. Children from commercial births are different from other children. Obstetrician-gynaecologists create additional pressure on neonatologists, especially if something goes wrong during childbirth]. I clarify, 'Are there two of you today (only two doctors)?' She replied that there were three of them, but one doctor had to be examining 50 children, and the second one couldn't get out of the maternity ward [since the beginning of the shift]. The midwife was standing in the corridor for a long time and was waiting for something. Then Dr. Lilieva quietly told me that paid-for rooms always asked her to conduct a checkup first. (Participant observation diary, maternity hospital, October 2020)

In the case of commercial childbirth, the need to provide emergency care to a newborn and hospitalisation in a paediatric hospital undermine expectations of safe and comfortable conditions and opportunities for parental control even more. Besides, such situations create a symbolic conflict between the maternity hospital staff and the resuscitation and advisory service, because the parties to the commercial contract try to maintain the image of well-being and well-provided services even in a critical situation with unfavourable prognosis:

> A doctor at the RAC gave an example of how she and a colleague of her were taking a child from a private maternity hospital. Her colleague told the parents that the child's condition was serious and he would be in intensive care for a long time. While the doctors of the maternity hospital told the mother, 'He just looks scary . . . because he's covered in wires (sensors), but later he'll get better

> and everything will be fine!' At the same time, they looked at us with such an expression (as if we were saying something wrong). (Participant observation diary, RAC unit, April 2021)

Thus, we have examined how a newborn patient can be considered as a unit of account in both 'paper' (bureaucratic) and economic dimensions. The work of the neonatal service is complex and complicated not only clinically but also in terms of the correct execution of all documents, which, not least of all, must take into account the material and financial provision of neonatal care. The next section examines another context that indirectly shapes the trajectories of newborn patients and the practices of health professionals – the sociopolitical one.

POLITICAL CONTEXTS SHAPING PROFESSIONAL PRACTICES

> Then [the neonatologist at the maternity hospital] says, 'He's good, though!' 'No matter he's not going to become the future president!' They keep joking that the patient may still be a presidential candidate and that perhaps their grandchildren will still vote for Bulgakov (the patient's last name). (Participant observation diary, maternity hospital, July 2023)

At first glance, medicine seems to be a depoliticised field in many contexts, and the work of medical professionals appears politically neutral. In the field under study, political issues were indeed not mentioned often, and were not clearly articulated by the informants. Political issues appeared mainly as jokes or informal discussions of the latest news from the media and political events that change the movement within urban infrastructures (e.g., international forums or the visit of the first person of the state). However, indirectly, some of the features of the political contexts, which the neonatology service was formed in over the past decades and continues to operate today, were also manifested in the daily interactions and practices of health professionals. This section describes and analyses those political features of the broader social context that, in one way or another, shaped the work of the care under study and the fate of newborn patients.

The shaping of the health system or its segments (e.g., maternity and newborn care) as influenced by government policies, occupational organisation, attitudes towards health technologies and their use have already been studied in other contexts, for example in North America and Europe (De Vries et al. 2002). Researchers have shown, in particular, that, on the one hand, the 'design' of obstetric care stems from existing political systems and cultural beliefs (see also Davis-Floyd 2004, 2), and, on the other hand, largely determines the experience of receiving assistance at the time of labour and birth, as well as the set of ritualised practices that constitute it (ibid).

When considering the political conditions, in which the healthcare system in Russia was formed and operates, it is important to mention at least two of its features. The first is that healthcare inherits both the design and regulatory logic of the Soviet system named after Semashko, which was characterised by high centralisation and dominance of state control (Field, 1957; Sheiman et al. 2018). The position of medical professionals in that system was considered bureaucratic, and the doctor was in many ways viewed as a literal state representative in the system of citizen-patient relations with the state (Field 1988; Saks 2015). A certain dependence of the medical professions in Russia on public administration and the statist direction of state policy in the field of welfare, including healthcare (Cook 2015; Matveev and Novkunskaya 2022), has a significant impact on the organisation of medical care and the way it is provided. For example, certain health care performance indicators become a matter of concern for the president of the Russian Federation and form the basis of so-called 'National Projects' – the federal policies aimed at solving certain problems. For example, starting in 2006, as part of the national project 'Health', the active construction of perinatal centres in many regions began, which significantly changed the infrastructure and design of obstetric care within the regions (including the routing of newborns) (Novkunskaya 2020). During the research (starting in 2018), several new national projects were also launched, including 'Health Care', which, for example, included 'reducing infant mortality (to 4.5 cases per 1,000 of born children)' as a target indicator (Passport of the national project 'Health Care' 2018).

The significance of such a target indicator for healthcare policies is determined by the second important feature of the political profile in Russia, that is, authorities' concern about the national birth rate. This characteristic of social policy is referred to by researchers as pronatalism (Rivkin-Fish 2010) and constitutes the second key feature of the political context of the field under study.

Researchers show that since the mid-2000s, social policy in Russia has begun to pay very close attention to issues of fertility, motherhood and childhood, as well as medical care in the field of obstetrics, including neonatology (Chernova 2013; Temkina et al. 2022). This attention is not only rhetorical in nature but is also reflected in the design of the reforms being developed, as well as in the organisational, infrastructural and practical consequences of their implementation. Examples of such pronatalist policies in the last two decades are the introduction of maternity capital (payments to families, which gave birth to the second and subsequent children; from 2020 payments were provided for families giving birth to their first child as well);

the introduction of a 'birth certificate', that is, a separate system of financing antenatal clinics, maternity hospitals and children's clinics, allowing women to choose a specialist for pregnancy monitoring and an institution for childbirth; as well as some measures to restrict access to abortions (in some regions, this is the adoption of the law 'On the prohibition of incentive to abortion' (see, for example, the Law of the Pskov Oblast 2023, the Law of the Kaliningrad Region 2023); as well as the introduction to the State Duma of the Russian Federation of a bill on banning abortions in commercial clinics (see Bill No. 510787-8)). The area under study, in particular, is affected by the symbolic embodiments of pronatalism. For example, it is the fact that the performance indicators of obstetric and neonatological care services are considered important indicators of the level of healthcare in general (Gonzalez and Gilleskie 2017) and become key performance indicators of political subjects (in regions and heads of regions). This section of the chapter examines exactly how those effects of government controls and policies are reflected in the work of health professionals and the decisions, which they make regarding the routing and treatment of newborns.

Management and Control

The above features of the political environment, which medical organisations and professionals operate in, are largely part of the discursive field, that is, rhetorical phrases of different political subjects, reflecting their concern about 'demography'. However, for informants, they are also part of a command and control system that shows how responsibility for newborn care is shared:

> Well, look, the story here is like this. . . . On the one hand, it is complex, on the other hand, it is very complex, thirdly, you are responsible for everything, but at the same time, of course, the requirements you have to meet are colossal. And if you understand that the infant mortality rate is one of the key indicators in general, and in our specific case [it is an indicator] of the work of Governor N., then, naturally, there is responsibility here . . . it is colossal, yes (sighing). (An interview with the chief freelance specialist of the region)

> Well, the procedure [of routing pregnant women] is generally very simple. Overall, it's simple because there are several stages, and it's like this – if the limits are exceeded, it immediately affects infant and maternal mortality. Right there. Therefore . . . [It turns out] that they will tear off head either for one rate, or the other. (An interview with a doctor-consultant of the RAC)

> I asked her [a doctor in one of the two neonatal intensive care units], who would deliver the foetus from the X-maternity hospital. Vera [the doctor] said that the child would be admitted to the fourth floor, that they [their floor] were full, and there were Kostya and Vitya [doctors] (up on the fourth floor) today. 'Let the

young people work, and we will improve the statistics', she said that calmly, but I think there was some kind of offense in her words. It is all due to the fact that the mortality rate is higher on the third floor than on the fourth. (Participant observation diary, children's hospital, September 2020)

Quantitative indicators of the performance of the neonatal care service are simultaneously an assessment of both medical departments and institutions and political entities, which has a double effect on the institutional structure of this field and the logic of its regulation. On the one hand, within the framework of federal and regional policies, many measures are now being taken aimed at creating conditions to improve those indicators. First of all, it concerns building the routing of pregnant women within regions in accordance with the degree of risk of complications of pregnancy and childbirth or fetal pathology that was diagnosed in utero. This system involves a comprehensive diagnosis of pregnant women, and based on results, each case must be sent to an institution of a certain level that has the appropriate technical equipment and qualifications of employees. Such a system allows, in most cases, to provide obstetric and neonatal care of the required level and volume (since the most complex cases are provided in the most equipped institutions with a high level of professional competencies), plus reduce maternal and infant mortality rates in the regions. On the other hand, the 'battle for numerical indicators' for political actors becomes an end in itself, sometimes divorced from medical and practical reality, where it is impossible to completely exclude deaths for both categories of patients:

> I have this, you know, mixed feelings. On the one hand, it is clear that when, back there, ten years ago, in general, in our country, yes, now we are talking about the country in general. . . . The number [of infant mortality] was much higher than now. Now, basically, in 2022, the country ended with a figure of 4.5 ppm [4.5 deaths per 1,000 live births]. Of course, this is very good, and it is very good that. . . . Figures are figures, but a huge number of lives have been saved, yes, throughout the country. They were saved as a result of the introduction of technologies for training personnel, both nursing and medical. There is the correct routing of pregnant women, already born children, and the building of perinatal centres [in the country]. I personally treat them differently and I will explain why. Across the country, again, there is a programme to build those perinatal centres. I mean this is all very good, but, on the one hand, we must understand that it [infant mortality] cannot reach zero. There is this desire to, though. . . . We cannot save all the children, but at the same time . . . (sighs). There is some kind of escalation of the situation, yes, of course. Well, this is generally typical for many issues in the Russian Federation. Our region, um, it is in the first, well, ten, or six, as it turns out. And the infant [mortality] figure,

> we had in 2022, was 3.4 ppm. Well, of course, this is 'better than' [expected]! (An interview with the region's chief freelance specialist)

Moreover, the race for good performance indicators, according to some medical professionals, turns out to be a form of additional pressure on healthcare managers and administrators, which, in turn, leaves no space for discussing medical ethics in each particular case, and even space for exercising the agency of families themselves:

> He [the head of intensive care] was talking about premature babies. In his opinion, parents of premature babies are in a worse situation, since they cannot decide to refuse resuscitation of their children and nothing depends on them. Later they suffer with those children, because almost all of them die or become deeply disabled. Meanwhile, the committee [the city's health authority] and the government are putting pressure on the performers to keep the mortality rates lower, forcing them to pull those children out [of the dead]. Although everyone understands that this is all for show. In pursuit of increasing the birth rate, they even dissuade women from having abortions (they deliberately delay gestational age). (Participant observation diary, children's hospital, March 2023)

It is worth making a remark that legislation and law enforcement practices in the field of resuscitation care in Russia leave virtually no opportunity to refuse resuscitation, even in cases with extremely unfavourable prognosis. The current methodological letter of the Ministry of Health recommends that neonatal resuscitation care be provided to all newborns, if indicated, who are born at a gestation period of ≥22 weeks and have at least one sign of live birth. Resuscitation in the delivery room can be provided to children without signs of live birth who were born at a gestational age of 36 weeks or more without anencephaly (Antonov et al. 2020). Thus, the only pathology, which neonatal resuscitation is not provided for, is anencephaly.

These features of the legal context of neonatology are discussed in detail a little late in this chapter. Here, it is necessary to consider how exactly the activities of medical professionals and organisations are controlled and how different regulatory logics compete with each other (Freidson 2001). It is important to emphasise that adherence to bureaucratic rules and political interests do not always outweigh professionalism as the logic for regulating the work of neonatologists and nurses. Such control over professional work is carried out by colleagues at different levels, that is, within departments, across a specific organisation, or even throughout the entire professional community, 'They didn't ask me about this at the hospital conference. The hospital conference has the function of control and, if necessary, of repression'. (participant observation diary, children's hospital, February 2020).

Within departments, control from management can be perceived no less painfully than from 'external' control and supervisory bodies. It is even more painful when this control is justified by distrust in the work of employees and calls into question their professional knowledge, experience and competencies. Even at the departmental level, management (heads of departments) may be perceived not as part of the professional community, but as external (and not always justified) supervision:

> Vitalievna (the third doctor on shift) is glad to see me. She pours tea and begins to ask about how things are going at the RAC, begins to complain about the frequent change of chief doctors in maternity hospital No. X, about the new head of intensive care unit named Galya. She resents having to report to her for [each child's] transfer. Olga [another doctor] arrives and falls into the conversation. She says that if she considers it necessary, she transfers children just like that [without reporting]. Olga mentions that she once transferred, and then she had to report back and 'it was unpleasant'. (Participant observation diary, maternity hospital, January 2020)

On the scale of the professional community, the heads of departments and heads of clinics can become objects of control themselves, first of all, by the chief freelance specialist of the region. As was shown in one of the quotes from an interview with such a specialist in the region under study, she [the specialist] is in many ways a mediator between the professional community and political entities (health committee, regional government); however, control on her part is often justified by ideas about professionalism and the most effective practices (in terms of clinical outcomes). In such cases, professionalism can be opposed to both sustainable (habitual) but ineffective practices of doctors and the logic of maximising economic benefits:

> Tatyana Yuryevna, the chief specialist of the region turns to me with a request and tells me a certain situation. Today she asked Alla (an RAC doctor) to check up how many hours the ventilator had worked in the transport incubator in the X-maternity hospital. She has suspicions that some maternity hospitals do not transport children in an incubator from the delivery room [to the intensive care unit], but carry them in their arms the old-fashioned way (this is true, according to my observations).
>
> [. . .] At the meeting, Tatyana Yuryevna raised this topic and explained the controlling actions on her part. She said that it had taken a lot of effort for her to purchase transport incubators, and she intended to make sure that they worked, 'My doctors photographed the hours (hours of operation) in your devices, I have this data on my phone. Now, when I come to you, I will be able to compare how long your ventilator worked during this time'. After the meeting, I go up to Alexandra again, we discuss something that was said on the podium, and

> then she says in all seriousness, 'You know, after that we started transporting children in the incubator, and we liked it. It only takes a long time, but it's so cool! They arrive so pink!' (Participant observation diary, professional conference, February 2020)

There are also the opposite situations, when experts or institutions endowed with supervisory powers reveal their limitations and professional insolvency. In such cases, experience and knowledge become a resource for resisting unjustified control and confirming doctors' professional status:

> A nurse tells another one that she was asked during advanced training about the principles of resuscitation, and she explained what to do first and what to do second, but she was told that she was wrong. She argued that everything was correct, though, because those measures should be taken up first with adults, and they are different for children. It was a story about success on the commission and how they [the professional development commissions] are unreasonably organised. (Participant observation diary, children's hospital, January 2020)

However, if within the professional community (both on the scale of departments, organisations and larger structures), management and control are not only based, to a greater extent, on ideas about professionalism (as a logic opposed to market and bureaucratic), but are also the subject of discussion within the framework of negotiated order, then non-medical control and supervisory authorities and inspections are most often described as completely external, often irrational rules that have to be taken into account in practical work, and which, in the event of the slightest violation, can lead to quite large-scale consequences:

> I notice the wrong headline in the header of the register – GBHI DGB No. X [state budgetary healthcare institution 'Children's City Hospital No. X'], but a few months ago our institution was renamed SBHI RHMADMC [state budgetary healthcare institution 'Regional Hospital of Medical Autonomy Districts and Medical Clinics']. After some time, the hospital received a large fine because the consents for treatment had had the old name of the institution in the headline). Then I wrote a message to senior paramedic Dmitry and warned him about possible problems. He took it calmly, but I remember us rewriting the registers for the whole year due to smaller errors (alright, my job is to warn). (Participant observation diary, RAC unit, December 2019)

Such external supervision makes control within the professional community be redefined in terms of professional learning, solidarity, and the general goal of minimising the possible costs of imposed external sanctions:

> A head of neonatal intensive care comments [at a conference of regional neonatologists], 'The conversation about mistakes cannot be limited to one time. Do you know what a colossal amount of attention is now paid to documentation and papers?' He continues, 'Our task is not to punish anyone, but to teach everyone how to get it right, so that later some external people cannot find fault and punish us, so that we are not set up and risk!' (Participant observation diary, professional conference, November 2023)

It is worth noting that quite different organisations and state bodies can be agents of sanctions, external to the professional community in the field under study, for example, insurance companies that check the correctness of medical documentation and have the right to fine medical organisations, control and supervisory bodies like Roszdravnadzor or Rospotrebnadzor, various branches of the executive authorities (city, regional and federal governments and ministries of health), and even law enforcement agencies (prosecutor's office, investigative committee). A large number of these regulatory bodies and authorities, as well as the contradictions between the rules they prescribe, create conditions for multiple vulnerabilities of medical professionals, who constantly feel as if they are objects of external control and possible sanctions, and at the same time do not have sufficient resources for self-defense (Litvina et al. 2019). The legal dimension of this vulnerability is discussed in more detail in the next paragraph, but it is important to mention here that they create conditions in which responsibility for decision-making sometimes becomes not part of professional work, but unwanted risks that professionals try to avoid. In other words, negotiations on the routing of newborns and decisions on their observation and treatment sometimes resemble a game of 'hot potato', when the desire to relieve oneself of responsibility for the future fate of a difficult patient becomes the key logic of the work:

> I explain the situation regarding the transfer, 'since the child is stable and we have problems with places in X- and XX-children's hospitals. It would be nice if he stayed with you [in the maternity hospital] until tomorrow.' At the same time, I'm trying to clarify, when he was born (how old he is). The doctor says that he is two days old, and she would like to transfer him today, of course. (Participant observation diary, maternity hospital, January 2020)

Responsibility for a critically ill newborn can be (re)distributed both between different sectors of care (and, accordingly, different medical organisations) and within one institution between specialists of different profiles. This conflict of interest between obstetricians-gynaecologists and neonatologists has already been discussed above, but it is important to mention that tensions and attempts to transfer responsibility to another person can also arise in the relationship between medical and nursing staff:

> U1.: Well, there are just some nurses, who, well, for example, there are some nurses, yes, roughly speaking, whom the doctor won't say anything, because he will immediately get an answer, right? And there are those, whom, yes, they can really rot, and well, it's just that, since I work as a head nurse, I sometimes have to. . . . Yes, well, because doctors often like to shift [responsibility] there, 'Why isn't this ready? It's the nurse's job'. The nurse doesn't care, because it's your responsibilities [as a doctor], you have to examine everything and make sure that you should have this, this, and this. Then you can say, 'Bring me this and that'. And this shifting [of responsibility] happens quite often.
>
> U5.: The last shifting that I had looked like this. The head of the unit called and said that a nurse, a nurse with just a basic professional education should read the doctor's diary. Because at the end, the doctor writes the prescriptions and she has to read them. I say, 'Wait, the nurse has a prescription list that she directly works with, and the doctor must write the prescription in it, and she works with this sheet all day long'. He says, 'No, she should read the diary, too, because the doctor prescribes in the diary, but may not write about it on the prescription sheet' [. . .] [it means] a nurse cannot forget something there or do anything else wrong. We have no room for error. And it was not possible to overcome this system, so the nurses read the doctors' diaries, making notes that they canceled the prescription. Yes, they confirm they are aware of the fact that they have withdrawn the prescription. I mean, well, this is a very sad story. (The focus group with nurses from maternity hospitals and RAC)

Responsibility and opportunities to delegate or avoid it are built into complex professional hierarchies within the field under study. These hierarchies are in some cases formalised in the relationship between the manager and subordinates (for example, the head and employees of the department, the head physician and the heads of departments), but sometimes different hierarchies and statuses within them are fixed in informal agreements. Arguments in such agreements can be not only different symbolic statuses (e.g., greater professional expertise and experience) but also uneven distribution of resources:

> [I hear them] discussing whether they will transfer [the child to a transport incubator]. As a result, Arthur [a doctor of RAC], after consultation with the main specialist, decides that he needs to wait about an hour for the child to stabilise, and then transfer him. They also need to wait for test results. He [the child] is not yet transportable. Arthur is explaining this to the head of unit for a long time, she tries to explain to him in turn that the child needs to be transported. He doesn't exactly argue with her, but persistently explains, again and again, that the child is not transportable yet and needs to wait. Then he consults with

> the chief specialist of the region (it turns out that in the end, in severe cases, she makes the decision, doesn't she?) Does it mean that Arthur isn't sure that he's ready to take responsibility? [The whole conversation is] like sort of bargaining. The maternity hospital personnel say that something could break there 'suddenly. And they won't give us much fentanyl!' They look at the tests. Things are getting better. It is the maternity hospital personnel, who say that it's better, 'He's actually become super!' (Participant observation diary, maternity hospital, January 2020)

It is the need to route a newborn in critical condition that often reveals such a discrepancy between the formal status of the institution or specialists and the real opportunities to provide the necessary neonatal care. For example, the regional routing system assumes that perinatal centres are third-level institutions that have the necessary equipment and qualified specialists to provide medical care in the most complex clinical cases. However, in practice, not all regions have the necessary resources even at the level of perinatal centres, and in some cases, the task of providing neonatal care in the required volume not only reveals a discrepancy between the actual equipment and the formal status of the institution but also goes beyond the formal routing system within one region:

> [This] child is extremely difficult. We are discussing that his transportation is not advisable. The doctor at the Perinatal Centre [of another region] says that she would like to transfer him, but this is impossible. [The motives and logic of the transfer are to get rid of a difficult child. The argument is the absence of a surgeon.] I agree with her, with another argumentation, 'We can transfer him, but does he really need it?' She tells me that he has burns, and they do not have a permanent surgeon, only a consultant, who comes two times a week. We return to the staffroom, I look at the tests and call Tatyana Yuryevna [a doctor], telling her that the child is extremely difficult, but I don't see the point in transferring. She asks me more about his condition and says, 'if this were our maternity hospital [region in which the RAC formally operates], would you take him?' I object, 'This is not a maternity hospital, it's a perinatal centre!' To which Tatyana Yuryevna replies, raising her voice, 'What kind of perinatal centre is this, [if there is no even surgery there]?!' (Participant observation diary, Perinatal centre, March 2020)

From the few pieces of data above, it can be concluded that the maternity sector of the neonatal care system most often tries to 'shift responsibility' for the patient to subsequent stages. As a rule, this is due to a lack of technical and professional resources, as discussed above. But in some cases, transport sector employees initiate transfers themselves, not trusting the qualifications and experience of maternity hospital employees:

> At about 21.00 we went to X-maternity hospital. When we were going up in the lift, I told my nurse that I didn't know if we would take the child. Smirnova [the nurse] said, 'Why should we wait? We have to transfer him, that's all!' I replied that not everything was so simple and sometimes it'd better to leave him in place. . . . She replied, 'They'll get him down to death, it's better to transfer!' (Participant observation diary, maternity hospital, October 2020)

Distrust of colleagues may also arise during further transfer of the patient, that is, already in the paediatric hospital sector. This is usually due to differences in professional practices and approaches to treatment, but also to a lack of material resources, since medical care for patients in the most critical conditions requires not only the highest medical expertise but also complex technical devices, which are limited in number and availability:

> After we transferred the child to their ventilator, difficulties arose because the device did not provide the required pressure (omissions of therapists, who usually prepare a place for a new patient). If the child had been in serious condition, I would have rolled back my transport incubator, which, by that time, the nurses had already rolled out into the corridor. But the child continued to breathe spontaneously, and at that time the therapist had already managed to roll in another ventilator. It is very unpleasant, when such hitches happen. This is a problem of succession in the treatment of the patient. When you try to do everything correctly and hand the patient over to the next doctors (from the maternity hospital you transfer him to the doctors of the RAC, from the doctors of the RAC you transfer him to the resuscitators of the hospital, and even carry him from one doctor on duty to another), often a feeling of mistrust or, in situations like this, a feeling of dissatisfaction and discontent arises. (Participant observation diary, Children' hospital, October 2020)

This section has shown how the political environment, where neonatal care is provided, can influence the professional practices of doctors and nurses, and how the different combinations of professional and managerial logics of governance create a complex system of responsibility for the patient and his or her routing. However, this dimension of the life of a newborn (his or her high symbolic value both in the categories of professional success and in the performance of the executive branch) is not the only manifestation of external sociopolitical conditions in the trajectory of his or her treatment. Another important dimension of neonatal care is the legal environment, including both legislative norms and features of law enforcement practices in this field.

Patient and Medical Care in Legal Categories

The normative-cultural approach to the study of organisations and the legal contexts in which they operate considers the latter as a system of moral principles that provide normative and cognitive guidance (Edelman and Suchman 1997). In such a theoretical perspective, organisations are viewed as parts of a complex institutional field or as specific positions in a socially constructed cultural reality. The law can form different environments for these organisations, that is, intermediary, regulatory and constitutive. Following this analytical tradition, the legal context of the existence of medical organisations is further considered as the conditions that embed those organisations in certain institutional hierarchies and clearly regulate their relationships. This constitutive legal environment sets down the defining categories for the organisational field. These basic typologies provide labels, categories and default rules for organisational behaviour that are taken for granted (Ibid: 484).

Medical law and legislative regulation of healthcare as a whole are not formally a key dimension of control over the work of medical professionals. As described in the previous section, professionalism and medical ethics are equally significant sources of formal and informal norms and rules that ensure the most effective and appropriate ways of providing care to patients. However, law and law enforcement represent a very influential way of regulating the relationship between doctors (and other medical professionals) and patients (and their relatives), which were largely formed to protect the rights and interests of the latter (Goold and Herring 2018; Borozdina et al. 2022). In practice, legal norms and potential practices for their application are updated not only at the time of legal proceedings but also in the process of work, when medical professionals, on a daily basis, independently determine whether their actions can become the basis for a claim on the part of the patient, and how they can justify themselves in the case of judicial proceedings, making certain clinical decisions (Borozdina et al. 2022, 200).

Thus, if the legal environment of neonatal care in Russia is considered as constitutive (according to Edelman and Suchman), then it is worth mentioning several of its features that set down certain standards of work for medical organisations and professionals. The first such characteristic is the accusatory bias (accusatorial bias), which distinguishes law enforcement practices and judicial decisions in the criminal law of the Russian Federation as a whole (Paneyakh 2014; Solomon 2018). The second feature is the increased attention of security and law enforcement authorities to the field of medical care, in particular, the chairman of the Investigative Committee, who is trying to criminalise medical errors. He has already ordered the creation of a separate department within the structure of the Investigative

Committee that would deal with iatrogenic crimes (Mustafina-Bredikhina 2017, 168).

At the moment, there is no notion of 'iatrogenic crimes' as a legal category in Russian legislation. Nevertheless, the number of criminal cases brought against medical organisations or their employees is increasing, not least against surgical specialists (including obstetrics and gynaecology), as well as anaesthesiologists and resuscitators (Gorbachev et al. 2020). The main articles of the Criminal Code of the Russian Federation, which are most often charged against medical workers, are Art. 109. 'Infliction of death by negligence', Art. 118 'Infliction of grievous harm through negligence', Art. 293 'Negligence', art. 238 'Performance of work or provision of services that do not meet safety requirements' (Mustafina-Bredikhina 2017, 169).

The case of a neonatologist from Kaliningrad, Dr. Elina Sushkevich, illustrates the influence of those features of the legal environment on the work of doctors quite clearly. In 2022, she was sentenced to nine years in prison for killing a newborn (according to the prosecution) by intravenously administering a lethal dose of magnesium sulfate to the child (it happened in the autumn of 2018). As we lack legal expertise, we are not in a position to evaluate the legitimacy of the accusation and the validity of the court's decision. It is not the purpose of this study to establish a cause-and-effect relationship between the actions of the accused doctors and the (fatal) outcome for the patient, but it is worth trying to briefly present the arguments of both sides (prosecution and defense), relying on open sources in order to show what rational argumentation they use and how the logic of the work of neonatologists-resuscitators is represented, and what symbolic consequences for the field under study the decisions taken lead to (both legal and cultural).

Here is how the chronology of events and the rationale for the clinical decisions of Dr. Elina Sushkevich and her colleague from the maternity hospital, obstetrician-gynaecologist Dr. Elena Belaya, are presented in the investigation version:

> In November 2018, a woman gave birth to a very premature baby, weighing 700 g, in a maternity hospital. Acting chief physician of the maternity hospital Dr. Belaya, having received information from the doctors on duty about the birth of a child and his serious condition and realising that the subsequent most likely fatal outcome of his life would worsen the medical statistics of the maternity hospital, which could negatively affect her further appointment to the position of chief physician, and also wanting to save money resources of the maternity hospital spent on maintaining the life support of the newborn, [she] decided to kill the newborn. To commit the murder of a minor, Dr. Belaya attracted Dr. Sushkevich, who arrived as part of the resuscitation team to provide medical

> care to the child and further transport him to the perinatal centre. (Investigative Committee of the Russian Federation 2019)

From this text, it follows that the deceased child was born extremely premature and, even according to the investigation, had a most likely fatal prognosis, but the severity of his clinical condition was not considered as the main reason for the clinical outcome. The doctors themselves, in describing their actions, are prescribed as persons, following an exclusively bureaucratic logic of work, who consider the medical statistics of the maternity hospital to be a priority over their own professionalism. Another feature of the investigation (prosecution) version in this case is the wording; that is, the provision of medical care is interpreted in terms of deliberate murder (by prior conspiracy) instead of a tragic coincidence in work, inevitably associated with the risks of perinatal losses.

The conviction caused clear criticism from the professional community (Volodin 2020; Di Renzo 2020), as unfounded from a medical point of view, incredibly tragic in its consequences for the fate of the particular doctor and also indirectly affecting the practice of the entire medical community since this case revealed priority accusatory enforcement over the characteristics of complex clinical work. Dr Elina Sushkevich was supported by both the general professional community (RosBusinessConsulting 2020) and eminent, high-ranking doctors, such as the author of an open letter in her defence, Nikolay N. Volodin, MD, Dr Sci Med, Professor, Academician of RAS, Honored Doctor of the Russian Federation, Head of the Pediatrics Department, Dmitry Rogachev National Medical Research Center of Pediatric Hematology, Oncology, and Immunology; President of the Russian Association of Specialists in Perinatal Medicine (RASPM), Moscow, Russia. In particular, medical professionals suggested (in their letter in support of Dr Elina Sushkevich) to take into account the symbolic effects and impact of this case on the field of medical care as a whole as well:

> Nowadays, doctors providing care to newborn children throughout our large and powerful country are discouraged, depressed, and practically devoid of faith in justice, the desire to work further, because it has become dangerous to the life, freedom, and health of the doctors themselves and their loved ones [. . .]. The citizens of our country will suffer the greatest shocks if an innocent doctor is cruelly and unfairly punished for a brave attempt to save the life of a child, whose survival throughout the world remains a miracle to this day, despite the development of medicine and technology, unfortunately. Trust in doctors will be undeservedly undermined, and the doctors themselves, out of disappointment and fear, will stop believing in their profession and leave it. (Russian doctors wrote a letter to Putin in support of the neonatologist Sushkevich, RosBusiness-Consulting 2020)

This letter clearly expresses not only support for an unfairly accused colleague, but also concern about the position of doctors in the legal environment of Russian healthcare in general, that is, their defenselessness and even fear of possible law enforcement. The discussion of the Dr. Sushkevich case could not have been mentioned and left behind the pages of this manuscript, without giving it greater importance when describing the features of the legal dimension of the work of neonatologists in Russia. However, in this study, there are a number of empirical data with a constant mention of this case as a source of fears about potential legal liability and the peculiarities of law enforcement in Russian healthcare:

> After the conference, the doctors and I discussed an article about Elina Sushkevich, in which witness testimony was published about how Sushkevich, on the instructions of the head doctor of the maternity hospital, administered a lethal dose of magnesium sulfate to a child. We couldn't understand how this was possible. Why [did she] engage in such forgery, when the team was ready to take away that child [from the maternity hospital]? Also, the statistics [mentioned by prosecutors], as it seemed to us, have nothing to do with it, given that this is a premature baby and the maternity hospital is not responsible for the cause of early birth. (Participant observation diary, professional conference, September 2020)

Features of legal regulation and law enforcement in the field of medicine in Russia are described by the informants, at times, as the main difficulty in the work of doctors and even as the key reason that not everyone is ready to remain in this profession. In particular, informants emphasise the injustice and inhumaneness of the judicial system, since it (according to them) is not based on reliable facts, creating incorrect interpretations of certain actions of medical workers, while remaining insensitive to their own vulnerabilities:

> I mean a very small percentage of people [out of the informant's 175 course mates] went on working in medicine. [. . .] A lot of people left, a lot of people quit, and this is due to the fact that, of course, Mr. Bastrykin [the head of the Investigative Committee of the Russian Federation], of course, did everything to show that medicine is so criminalised that somehow. . . . I don't really want to go to prison. So many people left [. . .] so in general. . . . Even after I quit, I was forced to go to the court. Unfortunately, when you see that it is black, and they tell you that it is white, then it is completely useless. This judicial system . . . you can't break it. The poor woman, yes, 58 years old, [she has a child, who is] already an adult, but disabled. Yet, she was imprisoned, though, and sent to a settlement in a colony. Of course, it's just terrible. I know a lot of such examples, and they appear to be convicted. Sometimes the statute of limitations expires, but still, it turns out that [even if] you are released in the courtroom,

> you have already been convicted. Formally. That's it, it's already a stigma. (An interview with a doctor-consultant of the RAC)

The above quote also shows that having a criminal record is not only a legal category or limitation for professional work but also a symbolic stigma. At the same time, informants emphasise that law enforcement does not take into account the peculiarities of medical care itself, in which, firstly, the lethal outcome does not always depend on the actions of doctors and nurses (the death of some patients is inevitable and unpreventable), and secondly, the assessment of the validity of those or other actions and measures taken is a complex task that lies in the field of professional expertise and which not all specialists possess by default:

> You know I work with experts from the Investigative Committee. Here I am working with absolutely amazing experts, as wonderful as no one [can imagine]. . . . There are actually very few of them in the country, as few as one can imagine. Every story, every case is analysed [thoroughly] there, [you can't imagine] how we discuss it, and so on. I mean it's worth a lot. Also, it's just very complicated. I mean it certainly shouldn't be that way, right? I mean everything should be sorted out and talked through at the level of medical organisations and medical experts. And this should be brought up [for discussion and analysis], you see, and not for punishments, birching with rods, right. I always answer, when, for example, they say to me, 'Your infant mortality rate has increased there!', I say, 'We don't kill anyone, right? That's how it happened. Over a short period of time [several newborns died] and that's how it happened'. And there [in the Dr. Sushkevich case] no one was killed. Well, this is nonsense. Even from the materials of the legal case it is clear that this is just some kind of nonsense, isn't it? And it's terribly offensive, it's terribly offensive, when you get involved into such things! (An interview with the main freelance specialist of the region)

The same quote from the informant shows criticism of the growing influence of the legal dimension on the work of a doctor. The control and regulation of medical professions in this perspective should remain within the boundaries of the profession itself and be the subject of error analysis instead of criminal proceedings. The number of criminal cases brought against health care professionals and organisations has been increasing in recent years, even though it remains quite low compared to some other contexts (for example, according to Jena et al., in 2011, about 75% of doctors aged 65, in the United States who work in low-risk jobs faced lawsuits, while this amount of doctors, working in high-risk specialties was 99%). However, the accusatory bias in decisions in the criminal cases gives the risks of such proceedings additional meanings, for example, fear of the inevitability of (unfair) punishment.

All this together creates an environment where the risks of legal proceedings are routinely taken into account in professional practices and negotiations, in particular, while drawing up the correct 'paper body' of the patient:

> I called the head of the paediatric intensive care unit at the hospital and told him about the child. He listened without enthusiasm and asked if it wasn't too early to transport such a child. I said that I agreed with him as a whole, but I would like to move him today, at least after 12 hours of life. We agreed on this. After that, Dr. Malvinova (she and Lyudmila were witnesses to this conversation) said, 'Here, Lyuda, just write down that the place was denied!' Then she added either 'for the prosecutor', or something like that. Eventually, the discussion ended up with variations on the theme that I would be imprisoned and Dr. Malvinova would be bringing me oranges and writing letters [while I'm in jail]. The situation was tense, as the maternity hospital really wanted to transfer the child. (Participant observation diary, maternity hospital, September 2020)
>
> Now, though, we seem to be more and more constrained [by formal rules], because there are clinical recommendations. . . . They, on the one hand, are sort of 'recommendations', aren't they? I mean you can choose 'whether you follow them or not'. On the other hand, for some reason, within the judicial system, they are perceived as mandatory! (An interview with a doctor-consultant of the RAC)
>
> U1.: Well, I can say that 25 years ago it was possible to write 'blood transfused' in the medical history, and forget it. I mean, you matched [blood type and Rh factor correctly], and that's it. Now, though, we need to fill in several documents, we have to meet a lot of conditions, and sometimes, it seems to me, we invent restrictions for ourselves, in my opinion, which are not provided for by the legislator. Over the past year, we've lost our minds about screening and consent to screening. This has generally become one of the most important documents in the history of the disease, although it is utter nonsense, and I am sure that the legislator, who wrote the law, did not even think about attaching such importance to this piece of paper. And for some reason, sometimes, in my opinion, we create unnecessary problems for ourselves . . .
>
> U4.: On the other hand, these papers are our security, too, some sort of protection from criminal prosecution, as well. (A quote from a focus group with doctors in the neonatal intensive care unit)

As can be seen from the last fragment of empirical data, such features of the constitutive legal environment cause not only a strict regime of adherence to formal rules, but also a sense of danger and personal (professional) vulnerability among medical workers. In the legal dimension, doctors define their work as extremely risky, but, unfortunately, they do not see reliable ways to minimise these risks or mechanisms to protect their professional and civil interests in the event of litigation:

[We have] complete insecurity. When something happens, your doctor [in the department] will naturally be left alone with his or her problem. And all these lawyers there, for example, and so on, it's all a personal initiative, who you choose, who works with you, [it is usually the one, whom you pay money]. Well, okay, your colleagues chipped in there, once, twice, say, right? But you need to understand that this is still not funded in any way [officially], yes. And the hospital here, well, maybe can provide some support, but mostly this is a statement of facts. (An interview with the main freelance specialist)

As studies show, violations in the preparation of medical documentation can become a self-sufficient basis for initiating criminal proceedings against medical organisations or employees (Borozdina et al. 2022), but it is still worth emphasising that the key aspect of resuscitation care of newborns, which is considered to be the most 'dangerous' in the legal dimension, is the death of patients. It simultaneously forms the core of resuscitation care and also turns out to be professionally and ethically the most difficult in terms of decision-making. As the case of Dr. Elina Sushkevich shows, deaths become the main sources of risk for medical professionals. Features of the legislation (mandating resuscitation in almost all cases, without taking into account the favourable future prognosis) and symbolically high risks of law enforcement create special legal conditions, in which resuscitation of a child (and its correct documentation) cannot be a matter of professional decision:

I.: What does now primarily limit the doctor from asking this question to the parents [if they should resuscitate the child]?

R.: Law. Absolutely the law. We are obliged to save each and every one, no matter what happens. Today there is no working law on how to diagnose 'brain death' in a child, although after 2012, when Dmitry Anatolyevich Medvedev signed the law saying that we could do this, there were practically no precedents. Then what's the point? So, we got a child, who fell from the tenth floor, he has a liver, a heart, but no brain. Brain's dead. What do we do? We will put a tracheostomy on him and feed him with a gastrostomy. Later, we'll tell his parents that we would love to turn him off, but, unfortunately, we will be sent to prison for many years if we do so.

I.: And what about the parents? Don't they have the right to do that, either?

R.: Parents cannot do anything because if the parents initiate this process, they will be imprisoned. I mean it's like killing a person left in danger, sort of by the conspiracy of a group of people or I don't know, in general, this is criminal liability, in fact, that kind of thing. (an interview with the head of the paediatric intensive care unit)

In the interpretation of the informant-author of the above quote, parents also cannot exercise their agency on the issue of the need and advisability of resuscitation actions. In a sense, the child's legal entity symbolically outweighs his or her social status, clinical condition and professional position, relative to the latter.

(Geo)political Context

When writing about the sociopolitical entities of a newborn patient and the multiple political and legal contexts that shape the work of medical professionals in recent years, it would be tricky not to touch upon the topic of global politics and military conflicts. However, this topic requires several ethical and methodological caveats.

Regardless of our own political views, we are committed humanists and opponents of any violent action by any government or force. At the same time, however, we believe that our research participants may have different attitudes towards current (geo)political events and (war)conflicts. Thus, articulating certain political positions could cause additional biases in the process of empirical data collection and potentially provoke communicative conflicts.

Despite the fact that our empirical study was conducted quite far from the territory of the hostilities, since 2014 the neonatal service in the region of study has faced (in one way or another) several consequences of the war conflict in Ukraine. According to our informants, during this period, federal healthcare centres have been accepting children for treatment on a regular basis. These cases have included newborns who required high-tech care, which for obvious reasons could not be provided in their home regions. We could not ask our research participants directly about their attitude to military actions and the effects associated with them due to legal restrictions as well. In fact, there is a legal prohibition on any assessment of military actions taken by the Russian army or other military forces, that are alternative to the official one (Federal Law of March 4, 2022). Thus, ethically, considering the safety of our informants, we did not provoke (with our interview or focus group questions) their reflection on this (geo)political context.

However, we could not include in our analysis one of the important consequences of the current political circumstances, which directly relate to the field of study – the actual restrictions to international cooperation for doctors and scholars from Russia in the fields of medicine and science:

> On the contrary, we do our best to work in a modern way here! I mean we try not to prescribe any nonsense, 'fuflomycins' [drugs with unproven efficacy],

> and so on. [. . .] I used to go (for internship or study) to Israel, to Germany. . . . Well, while you study and travel. . . . There were these good beautiful years, yes, which everyone remembers, these 11–12th (2011–2012s), we used to just buy plane tickets and fly somewhere to Belgium, for instance. There we listened to a seminar for three days, walked around for three more days and came back [. . .]. At that point in time, communicating with the giants of Western medicine, who write books, corresponding with them, I generally believed that Russia was on the path where we were still a little bit away, just a little bit, and we would catch up with them, we would be directly integrated into this [international] system. Here, but [. . .] And I felt this [restrictions for international cooperation] for the first time very clearly in '14 (in 2014), when we went to America for a conference, but it just happened before [the change in the political status of] Crimea. Here. [. . .] And, understandably, that, there we went to have lunch with them. And they [colleagues from the U.S.] said: 'Well, there's Obama back and forth [. . .] that let's reform this 'Heart to Heart' project, yes, and then ours will come again, we will come, you will come to us, here . . .'. They [colleagues from Russia] said: 'Are you crazy or what, are you crazy?! It's impossible! The governors never give their consent to such projects. . . . It's a technology transfer [possibly recognised as high treason], basically!' And that's why, of course, it's no longer possible. Here. And I'm afraid that, due to all the things which are happening [at the moment], this is probably, well, for me, the most sensitive issue in terms of, well, it's humanitarian technology, isn't it? Unfortunately, this is the point we are going to lose once again. (Interview with the head of the paediatric intensive care unit, April 2023)

Changes in the country's foreign policy inevitably entail changes at all levels of neonatal and intensive care: economic, logistical and, subsequently, the material infrastructure. Although medical drugs and equipment were not officially a subject of international sanctions imposed on Russia, changes in the logistics of supplies, as well as their rise in price, may have caused some limitations in the supply of components for foreign medical equipment. We cannot verify the reliability of such personal estimates, but in the perspective of some of our informants, such problems appear to be quite topical:

> There were cases of concentrators failing as well (. . .). And under the conditions of sanctions, despite the promised 'parallel import', I want to say that worklife is becoming more complicated [. . .]. Due to the problem, due to the refusals. Failures in equipment, failures in consumables, failures in spare parts in equipment. And the equipment, I want to say, is very expensive. [. . .]. The supplier will not refuse, of course, it's due to a manufacturers' position. And this is so, if you take the ventilator there. . . . So, for this artificial pulmonary ventilation, which is invasive, we have 'Puritan 560', here it's [made in] the United States of America. Here. If we are talking about non-invasive mask ventilation, which was very wide-spread in the Covid-19 period, yes, then it's 'Philips'. Philips

> is also American [product]. So, the Philips. . . . At the moment we have been refused the Philips, we don't know how to deal with the situation. There is an alternative, Weinmann. . . . These are German. . . . But it is suitable only [for patients] over 10 kg. . . . While we have 5 [kilogramme patients]. A fairly large percentage of children, and we have an increasing [proportion of such patients] every year - children under a year old. (Interview with a doctor working in the palliative paediatric service, June 2023)

Changes in the material infrastructure of neonatal and resuscitation or intensive care, as well as restrictions on the possibilities for international cooperation, appear to be quite palpable effects of wide (geo)political processes on the actual practices of medical professionals. In particular, it alters their medical approaches, and, as a consequence, the way neonatal care is organised and provided. Thus, the history of neonatology, which we described in detail in the first chapter of the book, resembles a cyclical composition (rondo), but with opposite practical effects. In the late 1980s and early 1990s, neonatal medical care received a strong impetus and additional resources for development through various international programmes and emerging forms of cooperation. But currently, we are witnessing a kind of return to a political regime in which both international cooperation and technological or professional breakthroughs in medical care are severely limited.

Writing about the limitations of international cooperation, it is worth making an important remark: the political effects we have written about concern primarily the relations with certain countries, which are labeled as 'unfriendly' within the state rhetoric. However, cooperation with other countries may, on the contrary, quite successfully develop and even take unexpected forms. This will be discussed in more detail in the final section of this chapter.

NEWBORN PATIENTS ON THE MARGINS

Resuscitation and intensive care of newborns require very prompt decisions and actions on the part of doctors and nurses, their high professionalism, and, in certain cases, sophisticated technical support. In the most critical situations, as a rule, the importance of legal regulation, contradictions of formal rules and different social labels are reduced, as they literally 'bare' a patient to just his/her physical body, which appears to be in a clinically severe condition. But once the criticality of this condition is reduced, a patient begins to 'flesh out' their multiple social labels and entities – legal, bureaucratic and political. This process can simultaneously reveal a lack of the 'proper' components of the 'paper body' and pose additional economic challenges for both the medical organisation and the family of a newborn.

In what follows, we will examine in detail the challenges that arise from the lack of the right paperwork for the (extended) newborn patient, with a particular focus on the administrative and professional tasks that must be addressed to overcome them. In this analysis, we will primarily rely on the interview with the deputy chief physician of one of the largest children's hospitals in the region of study, as processing the necessary documentation and communicating with funds to compensate for the medical care provided comprise her official duties. Here, in particular, is the way she describes the main challenges for the work of the organisation arising with the medical care provided to foreign citizens:

> There are laws by which we work, and for me, the law is the law. Well, in short, we work according to the law, and it is right that we work according to the law, because our conscience is clear, and no one will reproach us for anything. So, foreign citizens who are temporarily on the territory of the Russian Federation have the right to . . . [medical care. But] are obliged, to begin with, any foreign citizen who is temporarily on the territory of our state is obliged to go and insure themselves and their children, to buy them a policy of voluntary medical insurance. [. . .] Since foreign citizens do not realise their obligation and do not purchase a voluntary insurance policy . . . [thus, additional tasks arise to find funds for their treatment].
>
> So, according to the law on medical care provided to foreign citizens on the territory of the Russian Federation, the budget of our city is the only source compensating for medical care [provided to foreigners without medical policy], because we do not have health care for free. We have nothing for free. We bill. So, we bill, and we do not have the right to direct patients to the cashier's office [foreign citizens to pay for medical care themselves], if the service is needed to eliminate the threat to life. That's what the law says: 'a life-threatening condition and the amount of services necessary to eliminate the threat to life'. Translated into human language, it means resuscitation or surgery for a life-threatening condition that ends anyway, sooner or later a life-threatening condition requires [further] continued inpatient care. If it's not life-threatening, then it's the parents' responsibility to pay for it themselves. (Interview with the deputy chief physician for administrative and expert work, October 2023)

Patients without the necessary completeness of the 'paper body' (first of all, without a medical policy of at least one of the parents), in particular, reveal a discrepancy between the strict formal requirements of providing emergency medical care for newborns and the lack of its financial support at the regional level. In such cases, the economic burden falls on the medical facility:

> Every year, the budget of the city from our taxes allocates about half a billion rubles, which it distributes among the medical organisations of the city in order to compensate the costs of medical services provided to foreign citizens who did not take care to insure themselves and end up in hospitals in a life-threatening condition. Do you understand? Half a billion of our taxes! I have just seen the order of the health committee, in which the count for our hospital was. That was 33 million [rubles], which we're running out of by mid-summer. There is no more money in the budget of the city [to pay for emergency care for foreign citizens]. And until the end of the year we are obliged to treat these children, to save them, we are obliged, you understand, it's normal. But no one can find more money in the city budget, and all this medical care is provided from our own reserves. (Interview with the deputy chief physician for administrative and expert work, October 2023)

The lack of a patient's medical policy (as a basis for reimbursement of hospital financial costs) is not the only difficulty hospital administration faces while organising and providing care for newborn patients with non-Russian citizenship. Such patients also require the creation of a proper 'paper body', albeit under different regulatory rules, which primarily focus on their migration status and relevant legislation:

> one of the duties of our department is to put on and take off the migration register, because we have been equated to hotels. If we have not put a foreign citizen who came to us for treatment on the migration register, the FMS (Federal Migration Service) fines us, with half a million [rubles] fine. It's very tough. And so, our staff member goes to the FMS every day at the same time, she assigns those who had been hospitalised to the migration register. First, we have to find their documents with flashlights, you understand, right? That's why they check all the documentation that comes in every day, like through a sieve. And then we have to trace that a patient checked out and take him off the migration register. In general, it's a whirlwind. (Interview with the deputy chief doctor for administrative and expert work, October 2023)

In addition, due to the lack of residence registration in the region under study, such patients cannot be integrated into formal routing, for example, if palliative care is required rather than intensive care. Such cases comprise not only economic challenges (because resuscitation care is expensive), but also tensions regarding the number of intensive care beds occupied, which also constitute a critical but exhaustible resource of the neonatal service:

> many years ago, probably about 6 or 7 years ago, we had three children [without the medical policy] lying in the neonatal intensive care unit, then we understood and the parents understood that these were children on artificial ventilation who would lie in the intensive care unit until their last breath. Parents were ready for any outcome, but our rules of medical care prohibit euthanasia [. . .]. And a day

> in the intensive care unit costs 30 thousand for the state, that you understand. [. . .] A month, roughly speaking, almost a million, right? And it's wrong, it's wrong when there are other children waiting in line in maternity hospitals [for a bad in intensive care unit], and we can't take these children, because if it were a city child [with residency], he would go through the procedure of recognition of palliative status, then transferred to a hospice, and in the future assigned to the home ventilator programme. [. . .] And in any case with foreign citizens it is unrealistic, because no one can move them to palliative care.and give them expensive equipment from the city budget. (Interview with the deputy chief physician for administrative and expert work, October 2023)

As our key informant on this issue continued in her interview, the routing of patients with foreign citizenship, the continuity between different stages of care provided to them and the associated costs are beyond the scope of formal and well-developed professional, organisational and logistical solutions. However, the need to elaborate alternative solutions is not very rare, and as a consequence, they require professional initiative, some creativity, and additional resources. Such resources are, for example, charitable foundations and representatives of ethnic or national diasporas. In particular, they are attracted to find funding for the continuation of the treatment of a newborn if this treatment has a favourable prognosis or for repatriation if the continuation of hospitalisation is assessed as unpromising:

> And if there is a child who is good, promising, but there are no medical services available for him there [in the country of residence]. If here we can provide care needed, but it is expensive, then I have a diaspora. [. . .] We have very good relations with them, so if there is a good child who needs help, charity funds help. During these years of work, you know, we already have familiar charitable foundations that help, there are diasporas that help. There is this Pamir Diaspora, for whom the consul is not a person at all, they do not honor the law, that is (. . .). And if I say it costs money, and it is worth it, they help us to collect it. And if they say: 'We want to give money', I say: 'Guys, you will give money, but there is no point. You see, I am not sorry, but it is useless, the prognosis for life is not favourable. You will collect money, pay two million to the hospital, the child will not get better. It's better to go home while he's transportable. Because you will pay money, and then after all you will pay for transportation in a zinc coffin, which is also very expensive.' (Interview with the deputy chief physician for administrative and expert work, October 2023)

Some of the resources that the hospital administration attracts to construct an alternative trajectory for a newborn patient are literally disciplinary measures. For example, they may approach the Office of the Federal Migration Service (FMS) to forcibly discharge a patient from the hospital:

> There were parents, whom I had to. . . . They did not understand what I wanted from them, I had to contact the FMS migration service immediately. The FMS explained to them that it would be better for them to voluntarily get a ticket, buy a ticket and fly away, rather than this whole story [with deportation]. Well, in general, we have different ways to negotiate with parents, yes. (Interview with the deputy chief physician for administrative and expert work, June 2023)

Sometimes, the involvement of various authorities and administrative resources to address the issue of a child's transfer from the hospital goes not only beyond institutionalised trajectories but also beyond state borders:

> I started to think, in fact, whether I should write a letter to the minister in sunny Uzbekistan, that we have some children lying in some hospital on the outskirts of Saint-Petersburg? And why not? They are their [citizens'] children. And let everyone work. And in those days, there were no consulates here at all. There was only ambassador in Moscow. And just like that, I made a decision over the weekend. I came, sat down, wrote a letter to the ambassador in Moscow. And a copy to Tashkent, to the [Uzbek] Ministry of Health. The letter was about one child, who could be treated at his place of residence on an artificial ventilation machine in his very simple Samarkand hospital, because his parents were from Samarkand. There is direct flight connection. And it happened, a miracle: they were apparently so surprised, let's say, by the audacity of my letter that they called me from the [Uzbek] Ministry of Health and then called me back from Samarkand with the words: 'Tell us what is with this child, we are going to fly for?' (Interview with the deputy chief doctor for administrative and expert work, October 2023)

The re-hospitalisation of patients with foreign citizenship becomes possible only if an entire infrastructure is created, which includes families of a newborn, medical professionals from different countries, complex organisational, technological and logistical solutions, as well as legal and documentary support. Synchronisation of all the corresponding multiple entities of a newborn (material, economic, social, legal) in manual mode reveals at least two characteristics of the system under study. First, the already well-established and regulated system of medical care has grey areas that require innovative and even informal solutions. And second, the formal and official boundaries of this care (including state borders) appear to be quite conventional and permeable:

> In short, in short, according to the law, nobody is going to fly for a foreign child here on a Boeing, on a 'blue plane', or a helicopter, and pay for it all from the money of the Ministry of Health [of another state], that is, they just don't have budgeted it. Therefore, the most correct thing to do was to talk to the parents,

> who understood the severity of condition of the child, who understood that sooner or later the child will die, they understood that they are tied to our city for an indefinite amount of time, and they themselves have already earned money and would like to return home. So, we negotiated with the parents that they buy plane round-trip tickets for our doctors, and we do not charge a ruble for the work [. . .]. In general, this is a very expensive 'pleasure'. And then your humble servant coordinated it, with the consulate, we got documents for crossing the border, we wrote letters to the Ministry of Health. That is, once we have tried it, we have already worked it out. Then there is a long coordination with the air carrier, because oxygen tanks or oxygen cushions are allowed for some, but not for others. Well, in general, all of this has already been thought out, and this is an additional option, including in my work, so that these children without any damage and losses fly home, where they are met at the airplane ramp by pre-prepared medical facilities that are waiting for them. (Interview with the deputy chief physician for administrative and expert work, October 2023)

In cases such as those described above, the multiplicity of entities of a newborn patient becomes even more visible and palpable. Challenges in the process of compiling a 'paper body' of a newborn patient without Russian citizenship may also arise in the case of families with a higher economic status. Families that have sufficient economic resources (e.g., those who have applied for surrogacy services) but lack legal status also fall outside the institutionalised trajectory of a patient's treatment. Surrogacy, as a type of assisted reproductive technology, is legal in Russia, although, according to some experts, quite poorly regulated (Tolstikova 2017). As a consequence, citizens from countries where the use of these technologies is prohibited (e.g., from China) can apply for this assistance in Russia. However, in some situations (e.g., if a child born with the help of such technology requires intensive care), the legal status of a patient also turns out to be problematic for the implementation of formal rules and routing:

> I asked if a neonatologist come to arrange her 'Chinese' [patients] (surrogate children of PRC citizens) she, said yes. I told her that the day before I had seen a whole ward of surrogate children, also Chinese, at the N. maternity hospital. We were transferring one of them on the 22nd day [after birth]. She asked: 'Why did they detain him for so long?' and then she started to answer herself: 'I have one Chinese here who has bled me dry – he did not gain weight, he sucked 30 [millilitres] only and that's it! I found some leucocytosis in the tests, I was happy and started antibiotics, but it didn't help! And representatives of the Chinese [the patient's biological parents] begged to transfer him to hospitals, as they would have problems with discharge. One time we had to look for a surrogate mother to ask her to take the baby from the hospital and give him to the biological parents.' (Participant observation diary, maternity hospital, October 2020)

From the data quoted above, it may seem that the mother of a newborn has a more definite legal status and a corresponding 'paper body' (at least because it is formed chronologically earlier – before the birth of a child). However, this is far from being the case all the time, since the 'paper body' of any patient is primarily predetermined by citizenship: surrogate mothers have Russian citizenship and corresponding civil rights, including access to 'free' medical care. In the situation with a newborn whose biological parents have different citizenship, or whose status as parents has not yet been fully formalised, the Russian citizenship of a surrogate mother becomes a resource for a newborn patient to successfully follow the necessary trajectory. In cases when a mother herself does not have this resource, her own patient trajectory may diverge not only from that of her newborn, but from the clinically indicated one:

> The mom [with foreign citizenship] comes out. She is very pale, looks weak. I note that she speaks Russian quite well, I ask her about her clothes and tell her that we are about to heat up the ambulance car and she will only need to walk a couple of metres outside, I ask her partner to bring her things to the hospital. It turns out that she has a jacket in the closet. Rodionova (RAC nurse) asks her, what kind of baby clothes she has to wrap her baby. The paediatric nurse comes over and Rodionova asks her for a blanket, as the mom doesn't have enough baby clothes with her. After examining the baby I go to the residents' room to issue a medical card. About five minutes later Rodionova comes and asks me to come up, as the midwife came and they [maternity hospital staff] do not discharge the mom. I go to the post – there is an obstetrician and a midwife looking at the mother's tests, she has haemoglobin 65 g/l [which is extremely below the reference value]. The doctor says that with such test results she cannot discharge a patient. But the mother has no money [to pay for hospitalisation], and she will write a refusal and not stay in the maternity hospital. I go to the resident's room and call Hospital XX to see if they are ready to take the mom. After I informed the doctor on duty that the mom was anaemic and asked if they would take her as planned, she asked me to hold on and went off to consult someone, after a minute she said they couldn't take a mom with such haemoglobin indicators. I continued writing the card, Rodionova came up and asked 'well?' I said that we take the child, and the mom is going home. I asked the paediatricians if it was normal that they discharged a patient in such a condition? They are not surprised – they say it's a common story there. (Participant observation diary, maternity hospital, November 2020)

As in the case of a postpartum woman with anaemia who, due to the lack of the necessary documents (health insurance policy), could not get into the medical care system even though she had clear indications for hospitalisation, some newborn patients may not get into paediatric hospitals either. This happens, of course, not due to a shortage of resuscitation beds, but rather appears to be an effect of the inconsistency between the resources expended on the necessary care, the expected outcome of its provision (clinical prognosis), and ethical notions (both on humanism in general and the ideals of the medical profession in particular). In the next short paragraph, we will touch upon the cases in which a newborn's 'exit' from the neonatal care system becomes possible due to the actualisation of his or her social statuses, in particular, that of a representative of another culture.

IN LIEU OF A CONCLUSION: A NEWBORN AS A PART OF ETHNIC CULTURE

Empirical descriptions of the trajectories of newborn patients with non-Russian citizenship are put here instead of a conclusion. Such cases most vividly reflect the multiplicity of the entities of a newborn patient, their social construction and cultural predetermination. The narratives of our informants themselves reflect that the social, political and economic dimensions of neonatal care have a significant impact on clinical and organisational decisions regarding the treatment and routing of a newborn patient. At the same time, their contextualisation is recognised, as norms (both cultural and legislative) and traditions governing neonatal care in similar situations, but in different countries, are not always the same:

> The level of medical care in our country and in their homelands, in their states, from where these parents came from to earn money, is incomparable. And morally, these parents, because of their Eastern religions. . . . There's a completely different philosophy of how to treat a child, how to treat health issues, and how to treat diseases that are incompatible with life. These are their national features, and I accept it, because it is their faith and their way of life. But nevertheless, we live in our country, and we have a different attitude to all these issues and other laws regulating the provision of medical care to children with diagnoses incompatible with life and with unfavourable prognosis. (Interview with the deputy chief physician for administrative and expert work, October 2023)

The need to repatriate patients with non-Russian citizenship may, at first glance, be perceived as the one dictated solely by bureaucratic and economic logic: the intention to reduce additional hospital costs and avoid the difficulty of attracting necessary funding for a patient without the proper 'paper body'. Nevertheless, in the informant's narratives about these cases, we also see the manifestation of a professional logic that takes into account the patient's clinical prognosis, on the one hand, and ethical aspects of care, such as humane treatment, on the other:

> Our doctors who accompany them – they are usually met there immediately, at the airplane ramp right with the ambulance car. They go from the airplane to these medical facilities directly, hand over the child, tell the doctors about all the details [on his condition], exchange contacts. And, accordingly, the parents live at home, the child is treated at the place of residence, and when the life ends naturally, because it is a little easier [to arrange] there than in our country, the child is treated without any autopsies, according to the laws of Sharia, Islam and whoever else you want, in a human way. . . . And grandparents will be able to meet the child, look at him alive, you know? And then, according to the laws of Islam, before sunset, he will get a grave, which relatives will be able to visit. The worst thing is when children die here, and there are these unmarked graves. This is not humane, in any tradition this should not happen. A child should be where his [relatives] are, you know? And he should be seen alive by his grandparents. It's very important humanly. (Interview with the deputy chief physician for administrative and expert work, October 2023)

The above excerpt from the interview is a bit of a contrast to what we described and analysed in the third chapter of the book, devoted to the social labels assigned to newborns. In that chapter, we particularly described ethnic labels, which reproduce the important symbolic distinction between 'us' and 'them' by marking culturally and bodily the 'other'. In describing cultural norms regarding death and dying, 'other traditions' are not presented by our informant as 'wrong', 'uncivilised' or 'incomprehensible', but, on the contrary, as most humane, in many ways contrasting with an approach patients would experience if they remained in the Russian system of healthcare. By collecting information about the patient's relatives, their religion, region of residence, and the social structure of the community, while elaborating on the patient's (cross-national) trajectory of treatment, our informant is essentially taking an anthropological journey of learning about another culture:

> So even here's this baby who's being brought in today, I don't know if they showed his photos to you or not? It's a severe genetic pathology with malformation of the entire bony component. And they [the patient's relatives] live, they are the most mysterious, they are Pamir Tajiks, who are not Tajiks, they are Pashtuns, they were just registered as Tajiks. This is the Gorno-Badakhshan region. This is like Afghanistan, and here is Pamir. These people live here, where they have no authority, they have a mullah in charge. Whatever the mullah says, that's how it will be. Do you understand what I mean? Vanj district, Gorno-Badakhshan Autonomous Region, Tajikistan, I've already studied it all on the Internet. I looked, I thought: 'Oh, my God, oh, my God! How will they treat him?' So, they will take him to a place where a mullah will read [prayer] to him, he will lie there for a little while, and then they will take him away, sing a dirge for him, and everything will be normal. You understand, right? And it's

normal for them. (Interview with the deputy chief physician for administrative and expert work, October 2023)

Social norms in this story reveal their contradictory and contextualised nature. On the one hand, the institutional order of intensive neonatal care in Russia is presented here as literally the one limiting the ability of medical professionals to follow a more 'humane' approach. This context is described as highly regulated, in which official rules and legislation may contradict both physicians' and families' notions of the interests of a newborn. In the case described above, turning to other cultural and institutional contexts allows healthcare managers and doctors to escape these strict norms and to create an environment in which legal regulation, tradition and the expectations of patient's relatives do not conflict with each other. In this process, the professional medical gaze deliberately de-medicalises (and de-objectifies) a newborn patient, and the professional work is directed not on the physical body and its clinical outcomes, but rather on a patient's social and cultural entities.

Conclusion

Turning to the multiplicity of the entities of the newborn patient in our study, we can hardly come to one simple conclusion. Multiplicity turned out to be not only a key characteristic of the empirical field under study and not only our analytical lens through which we looked at the newborn patient and the neonatal care, but it also characterised our methodological position and our results. The newborn turns out to be far more than just a long-awaited child for the family or a medical body to be manipulated. The little patient, who does not even yet have a personality and agency in the full sense, already appears in many entities and is involved in many contexts at once.

First, the baby's body becomes part of a socio-technical system: it is surrounded, literally braided, with equipment that needs to be purchased, customised, repaired, supplied with replacement parts. This requires specialists, financial resources, established supply channels, creativity, ingenuity in the field to compensate for missing parts. In turn, this material and social infrastructure does not exist as an objective given but has its own history of formation. In this history, the emergence of new technologies and methods of treating/nursing newborns sometimes becomes not a condition, but a consequence of professional agency. Thus, the newborn patient, the medical professionals who return or sustain his or her life, medicines, technologies, and other parts of the material infrastructure find themselves in complex relations of mutual influence and formation.

Second, we find that the newborn patient included in the neonatal intensive care system has at least more than one body – the need to keep accounts and medical records, thereby ensuring his or her routing and treatment – that creates what we have called the bureaucratic or paper body. This result adds to the discussion of the 'paper/file self' (Fitzpatrick 2005; Shevchenko 2023) serving as a kind of analogue of the individual to the state, which other researchers have written about. In the context we are studying, the document flow produces not a new personality but a new, paper, body or demographic unit – the unit of accountability. Without it, the patient is not viable within the bureaucratic system; the completeness of this body may, among other things, influence the trajectory of their hospitalisation and even clinical decisions. The paper body does not just follow the physical body of the patient, being its additional attribute, it can replace it, coming to the forefront both in the case of administrative decisions and in the treatment process, when doctors are guided by the results of tests or records in observation charts, without comparing it with the real physical condition of the patient. Moreover, in case of a patient's death, their paper body will continue to exist, being a 'participant' in inspections, clinical discussions and court proceedings.

Despite the extreme degree of medicalisation of the context under study, the newborn patient appears in it not only as a body with certain clinical characteristics and not only as a bureaucratic unit of account. Even here, where the infant may weigh hundreds of times less than the surrounding equipment or the incubator that sustains his or her life, there is space for personalised communication and 'social labels' that function as the interface through which multiple social relations and characteristics are reflected upon the newborn patient. In the interactions of doctors and nurses with patients, we find many examples of demedicalisation, such as the emotional dimension of professional communication, attribution of emotions, intents and character (like a 'fighter – not a fighter') to infants, gender stereotypes and construction of kinship relations (connections with the mother, such as 'think of a name, he will hear you', 'mom, don't cry'). Through such social labels, the patient is included in culture and society, and in some contexts, ethnic, civic and cultural statuses literally outweigh the medical parameters of the newborn. We also observed how even in an extremely medicalised and bureaucratised context, for instance, in the case of readmission of patients with non-Russian citizenship, the trajectory of (de)hospitalisation is built not in relation to the physical or paper body, but in relation to the infant as a carrier of a different culture.

Third, because the newborn patient is not an independent, self-sufficient person, he or she is augmented at the expense of the mother, parents and the family as a whole. When interacting with the infant, doctors and nurses in a number of contexts deal with the 'extended patient', where it is impossible not to take into account the mother's or parents' decisions, not to obtain their consent, and not to interact with them, explaining what is going on with the child. The 'extended patient' not only expands the set of suffering and vulnerabilities that are inevitable in the neonatal intensive care field but also creates additional challenges for the work of medical professionals. We analysed these challenges in the book in the categories of emotional work and, in particular, showed that in practice it varies significantly between different sectors of neonatal care (maternity hospitals, transport teams, neonatal intensive care and pathology units in paediatric hospitals), and different professional groups (neonatologists and nursing staff). Emotional work is done in different forms and with varying degrees of intensity, and the regulation or manifestation of emotions, both at the level of narrating and in direct interaction, appear to be tied to their understanding of professional identity. At the same time, emotional work often remains invisible and goes unnoticed, so it was for us to give voice to our research participants in this respect: for us, it is an attempt to pay tribute to them and an opportunity to respect the principles of reciprocity in sociological and anthropological research.

We would also like to recognise that we ourselves, as researchers, were not always able to keep our position and experiences neutral. The situations observed in the field were in many ways connected to our own emotional experiences – sympathy, regret, indignation, surprise and other feelings also became our analytical tools, allowing us to detect social tension where there seemed to be a stable social order. Our own emotional work during the empirical data collection process was somewhat similar to that of the medical professionals we studied – we controlled those feelings that could disrupt work communication. However, on the pages of field diaries and in discussing our observations with each other, emotions also helped in finding methodological decisions, in posing research problems, in interpreting empirical data and in formulating counterintuitive conclusions.

Finalising our argument on the multiplicity of newborn patient entities and the multiplicity of our research findings, we would also like to return, in a sense, to the 'multiplicity' of authors and the fact that for each of the authors of this book, the research journey has also taken different trajectories. Therefore, we would like to conclude by sounding like separate voices once again.

ARTEMIY

The research project on neonatal service, which at some point turned into a book, is a story that happened 'in spite of'. Initially, my interest in anthropology was in no way related to my work as an intensive care physician, but rather to a desire to do something completely different from my main job. I would even call it an attempt to escape from the profession. However, my co-authors convinced me that the study of neonatal care was promising, for which I am very grateful. My main motivation in this project was to show how the complex system of neonatal care in the region works and to find key points of improvement of this system, although initially, it seemed to me a perfectly fine-tuned mechanism. But as the project progressed and as I communicated with my co-authors, I was able to recognise that the perceptions and knowledge of a person deeply immersed in a problem are not always objective and complete. The idea of applying the results of the research quickly lost its relevance, and even the answer to the question of how it works, which initially did not even seem like a real question to me, hung in mid-air. Since our research group consists of a sociologist, an anthropologist and a physician, I will allow myself to depart from the scientific paradigm of humanistic sciences and still say a few words about the practical significance of this work, making my colleagues responsible for the more theoretical conclusions.

Not many doctors, at least in Russia, read papers in sociology and anthropology of medicine. All their free time is taken up by the actualisation of medical knowledge – clinical recommendations, fresh guides, accreditations and routine attestations. At the same time, medical ethnography could be a step in the direction of rethinking one's practices and looking at familiar things with fresh eyes and better understanding not only their patients (or the relatives of the patients) but also their colleagues and oneself. To be a professional is not only to know how to treat a patient but also to know how to interact with his relatives and colleagues and to understand how the system is organised as a whole, not just in a particular department. This knowledge is not just a part of outlook; it is a defence against misunderstanding, conflicts and 'burnout', whatever we mean by this term. The patient multiplicities we have described and listed above, which, among other things, for each stage of treatment acquire their own unique configuration, undoubtedly turn each clinical case into a unique one. But these are not mere words; practical benefits can and should be sought in this knowledge. For example, cultural differences uncovered by physicians in the process of readmitting patients help to cope with the psychologically difficult situation of actual termination of care. The use of labels actually creates an imitation of agency, giving the patient properties that are assigned to him or her externally by the health professionals themselves, a mechanism that underlies both medicalisation and demedicalisation. Awareness of these mechanisms can help avoid situations in which the self-created configuration of the patient leads to severe deviations in the patient's treatment trajectory or conflicts.

The project 'Birth of the Patient' is not only an opportunity to show a newborn baby as a universal model of a patient without agency but also a demonstration of how he or she acquires this agency or pseudo-agency. Using the example of a newly born person (patient), we see the specific type of agency, or, in our case, its simulation, that can appear exclusively within the framework of interaction within the medical system. By assigning certain qualities to the patients, medical staff themselves complicate the configuration of their patients, thus taking them outside the biomedical paradigm.

By showing the perspective of physicians working in different institutional settings in this paper, we have tried to find a vantage point that allows us to look at the doctor-doctor and doctor-patient systems from the perspective of an external observer, although my perspective initially implied introspection. I hope that this work will be useful not only for representatives of the humanities and social sciences but will also resonate with the professional medical community and become one of the tools for professional development.

ANNA

One of the first books read by students entering the anthropology department of the European University at St. Petersburg is *Ritual in Traditional Culture* by Albert Baiburin. Its section devoted to describing elements of Slavic birth ritual, which describes the child's gradual introduction to the social world, is called 'From Nonhuman to Human' (Baiburin 1993, 29–61). It is not enough for an infant to simply come into the world to be separated from the natural, non-human domain and to be included in the human world. It is necessary to carry out a number of procedures on the child: from cutting the umbilical cord, abluting, giving a name, baptising and so on, to 'opening' the child's organs (vision, hearing, ability to walk and speak). Thus, a child who, after all the rites have been performed, did not start to walk was considered a 'changeling', a representative of the other world, that is, not a fully human being. Weak, sick infants were subject to ritual 'overbaking' in the oven, in analogy with bread-baking, but according to some regional ethnographic data, all infants were supposed to be 'baked' and 'finished', because of the belief that they were born 'raw'.

We can hardly draw direct analogies between such ritual overbaking of a weak child and the work of modern resuscitators and neonatologists on a child lying in an incubator, although perhaps to a Martian, these actions would look somewhat similar. However, being an anthropologist, I could not help my interest in the question of how culture draws the boundaries between the human and the non-human. It was once with this question in mind that I set out to conduct my first fieldwork: in my dissertation research, I attempted to look at how this happens in relation to a severely disabled child living in a residential care institution. Different groups of people surrounding the child (the staff of the state boarding school and volunteers of NGOs) drew these lines in different ways. Representatives of these two different communities practised different techniques of symbolic inclusion of the child into the world of humans, or exclusion from it. Although this project is called 'The Birth of the Patient' and not 'The Birth of the Human', it became, for me, a logical continuation of my initial anthropological drive and quest.

In our case, the child is deprived of inclusion in the social world through the elements of modern birth ritual, as these elements are inapplicable: he or she is not carried out of the hospital with a pink or blue bow, the mother is not greeted with bouquets by relatives and no photographs are taken or posted on social media. In the case we are studying, doctors and nurses, who are responsible for the child's life in the first hours and days after birth, not only incorporate a newborn into the human world through the social and bureaucratic labels assigned to him or her, but also draw their own distinctions between these labels. Some of them are noticeable at the level of observation of direct communication: for example, a fairly stable infant with a favourable prognosis will be coddled and communicated with using the baby talk register, while a newborn in critical condition in all senses occupies a borderline status and cannot be included in the culture through such speech practices.

At the level of narration, physicians also actually distinguish a category of newborns on whom it is not quite reasonable to spend moral and economic resources, since they will not be able to fully enter the human world, or even the world of the living, and will spend their short life in a palliative status. However, the boundaries between human and non-human are completely challenged by children born with the most severe pathologies, who are destined to live for only a few days. These children are hardly interpreted by our interlocutors as human beings, and when they discussed the value of their birth, I could not help but think of a classic passage from Mary Douglas, despite the different contexts:

> When a monstrous birth occurs, the defining lines between humans and animals may be threatened. If a monstrous birth can be labelled an event of a peculiar kind the categories can be restored. So, the Nuer treat monstrous births as baby hippopotamuses, accidentally born to humans and, with this labelling, the appropriate action is clear. They gently lay them in the river where they belong. (Douglas 2003, 40)

The difference here is not only that the practices described by Douglas with reference to Edward Evans-Pritchard's materials regarding children born with developmental abnormalities now look inhumane or cruel and cannot be part of modern society. But it is also true that the birth of such children is no longer seen by our interlocutors as an accident, but as a medical error that could have been prevented.

It is also relevant to our context that the boundaries between human and non-human (child and 'foetus') are drawn not only in direct interaction with the patient but also through state legislation. In the last decade, with the development of medical technology, we witness such an expansion of the category of 'human', when newborns, previously considered foetuses, have become live births (i.e., children and full-fledged humans). Advances in science and biomedicine have made it possible to nurse and treat children born at a low gestational age or with complex pathologies. However, scientific and technological progress, and over-medicalisation as part of it, are not just incapable of completely eliminating psychological and physical suffering, but as philosopher and social critic Ivan Illich [Illich 1976] has shown in his famous essay 'Medical Nemesis', they create new suffering, vulnerabilities and pathologies, whether medical or social.

What is important in this picture is that this expansion, as well as the pursuit of preserving the life of an infant born with extremely severe pathologies, becomes part of the state's demographic efforts. In this way, the newborn, statistically becoming part of the 'world of the living' (or the world of human beings), embodies a political interest. The logic of over-medicalisation, dictated by both progress and the state logic of care, might simultaneously save lives and multiply suffering, leading to prolonged dying and severe disabilities. This, in turn, raises questions not only about what a human being is but also about what humanism and, conversely, dehumanisation are, and how these concepts are constructed by different actors and stakeholders in the field we are discussing.

In a certain sense, our research belongs to the tradition of dark anthropology and the anthropology of suffering (Ortner 2016). During the fieldwork or while analysing the materials, I personally felt the human suffering and vulnerability in many aspects so close to me that it made me suffer and feel vulnerable as well. It was personally difficult to distance myself emotionally from some situations, such as that of a mother whose last chance to have a baby after many attempts of IVF ended up in a premature birth with disabling pathologies and who will suffer for the rest of her life from social exclusion, lack of support and falling out of the 'normalised', typical life scenarios. Or, like that of the children born with severe disabilities who survive and are finally permanently placed in state-run institutions, including orphanages, when parents realise that they do not have enough moral or economic resources to care for them. As I conducted my first fieldwork in an institution of that kind, I could see that it would be a place of suffering for the child, as nobody would lull her or hold her in their arms there, just feed and change diapers. At the same time, our project is about hope as well, like in the stories of saving the child weighing 380g at birth, which is a triumph of medical professionalism and courage.

Another encouraging facet of the project for me was the work and interaction of our research team. I must confess I felt a little bit envious while watching the harmonious, coordinated work of the transportation crew, as being a part of such a collective is a true blessing. But while working on our research project, it seems, we managed to reach the same vibe. I felt support, understanding, and secureness, as I knew that there was always someone 'on standby'. Our project and teamwork, for me, turned out to be, in the terminology of William Reddy (Reddy 2001), a sort of 'emotional refuge'. I am deeply thankful to my co-authors, Asya and Artem, for this experience.

ANASTASIA

This research, embodied in the book, has become (or has always been, as it seems now) more than just a working project with a predetermined research question, a developed methodology and a set of empirical and analytical steps. The irony is that we met Artemiy just as we, together with Anna, were delivering a course on qualitative methods, discussing with the students all these mandatory elements of research design, the ethics of qualitative research, and basic methods of data collection and analysis. It seems that little of the original idea remains in this project, and I must admit that as a sociologist and a teacher of qualitative methods, I have failed in many ways: I cannot articulate one clear and original research question that would guide our methodological steps, I cannot reconstruct one consistent conceptual model, some of the interviews and observations conducted did not follow a pre-designed guide or rubric, and the original hypotheses turned out to be irrelevant to the field. In general, however, I consider it both a professional and personal good fortune how this project turned out in the end, how my own social roles changed in the process of its realisation, and how our relationship with Artemiy and Anna developed.

In my final statement, I would like to talk about this book as a long research journey in the field of neonatology and as an amazing adventure in which I made real friends, and a little bit about how many intersections happened between the plot twists of our book and my personal biography. I hope the reader will also find something in it that touches him/her personally.

So, as a sociologist of medicine, I became acquainted with the field of neonatology long before I met Artemiy. My master's thesis and then my doctoral dissertation were devoted to reproductive health and the system of obstetrics in small towns in Russia, and initially, the key informant in this field was my uncle, a neonatologist working in a small town. When I went to work with him, or just to meet or get acquainted with informants, I did not go into the rooms where there were newborns, as if children's crying marked a certain sacredness of the space – the space where life is born and where I thought my own presence was inappropriate. Then I visited many different maternity hospitals, including perinatal centres, where I, afterwards, together with my colleagues Anna Temkina and Daria Litvina, observed the work of neonatal intensive care units and saw babies, including those born prematurely, quite closely. The field of neonatology became a little less sacred but still not literally a subject of research interest.

I found it interesting mostly because of its symbolic load – I was constantly reading the news discussing political decisions in regard to childbirth or the work of neonatologists. I was very moved by these public discussions, and on July 1, 2019, I even added a badge to my social media profile in support of Elina Sushkevich – five years later, even with all the political events that have taken place, this criminal case still seems to me one of the most unfair and dramatic in the history of Russian law enforcement. That same year, we recruited students for the Social Studies of Health and Medicine programme, and as part of a required course on qualitative methods, we met Artemiy. Initially, Artemiy wanted to study the field of psychiatry, but Anna and I, as well as Artemiy's coursemates, were so fascinated by his stories of working as a neonatologist that we eventually collectively deployed his own and research interest in his professional work. Artemiy's diaries, already when he was a student, seemed incredibly interesting, as if they were windows into a parallel universe where saving someone's life is a daily routine.

In the same academic year, a pandemic broke out, all of our own research fields were closed, and Artemiy continued to keep diaries of observations of the dramatically changing medicine, and through it seemed that I kept in touch with the empirical field I already loved. Then, in 2021, Ekaterina Borozdina and I became editors of a special issue of the Journal of Social Policy Research, where Artemiy was invited to write an article based on the results of his graduate work. Anna and I became co-authors of this text to help it fit into the framework of a 'sociological scientific publication', and we were terribly disappointed that this framework was so rigid that the wealth of empirical data seemed to be lost. So when, by chance, the idea of writing a book came up, we jumped at it together as an opportunity to show how much more interesting things (both empirically and sociologically) were happening in neonatology. And this was how this collaborative research adventure began. I am proud of how much we have done in the process of gathering empirical data about neonatology: that we have been able to talk to those who were at the roots of establishing the service when the field of medicine itself did not yet exist, that we have been able to gather and conduct focus groups with doctors and nursing staff. I consider it an incredible stroke of luck for me as a sociologist to be able to be in the spaces of observation that I have been in during this research. But what I appreciate most about this research is how our team came together, how we learned to discuss different issues (both empirical and analytical), albeit from different perspectives, in the same language, and how we developed not only a whole book but a true friendship as a result of our work.

And while I know that it is not customary for researchers to share much about themselves in the scientific literature, I will still allow myself to share how my own social positions and roles changed over the course of this study and book. Almost at the same time that Artemiy began his observations as a neonatologist as part of qualitative methods class, I learned that I was pregnant with my second child. My son was born three days before Artemiy's thesis defence, and as I was giving my feedback as his supervisor, he was also giving his voice as a newborn baby. At the time, we joked that neonatology doesn't leave Artemiy even at the defence, and my son and I ensured that all members of the examination committee were immersed in this experiential field. Six months after that, in the spring of 2021, my father got cancer; a few weeks before his death, we learned of my mother-in-law's cancer, and a week after her death (in late 2023, when we turned in the first draft of the entire book manuscript), multiple hospitalisations, including hospitalisation into the intensive care ward, of my father-in-law began. Thus, the issues of birth, life and death over the past four years have become not only the subject of my research interest but also of my personal experience. Not all dimensions and components of this experience I can rationalise – many of them remain exclusively in the realm of emotional experience. But at the same time, I think that some twists and turns of personal biography have also helped me in my research work, while empirical stories from the field and our analytical pursuits have, on the contrary, supported me in situations of living personal loss. Perhaps, in addition to contributing to the social studies of health and medicine, it might be a support for someone in the contexts and within experiences where the proximity of life and death can be frightening and difficult to explain and rationalise.

Appendix 1

Guide for Expert and Biographical Interviews with Medical Professionals Involved in the Institutionalization of Neonatology Since the Late 1970s

INTRODUCTION

Good afternoon,

We are researchers from the European University at St. Petersburg, and we would like to invite you to participate in a project on the history of the formation and organization of neonatal care in St. Petersburg. We wanted to learn about your experience in neonatology, your professional biography and peculiarities of neonatal patient care.

The study is supported by the Associated Professorship on Qualitative Health Research and is conducted in compliance with all ethical standards of social research. Your participation in our project will be anonymous, nor will we disclose your place of employment or other personal data or confidential information. The results of the study will be presented in a summarized form and used for educational, research and scientific purposes only.

If you still have any clarifying questions about the methodology or ethics of the research, you can ask them now or at any stage of the project [researcher's contacts]. You may also refuse to answer any of the questions asked and withdraw your consent to participate in the study at any subsequent stage until publication.

We ask your permission to record our conversation for transcription – Do you consent to an audio recording of the interview?

Background Information

How did you decide to become a doctor? Where did you study?
In what year did you start working?
How did you come into the specialty (neonatology)?
In which institutions have you worked? What are the stages of your work as a doctor? What is your background in the profession?

Neonatal Care before the Institutionalization of the Service

What did you do before the specialty was institutionalized (officially since 1987)?
Who and how were newborns cared for in maternity hospitals and hospitals when you started your work?
Did you have experience with premature babies?
What was the legal and medical status of premature babies?
What were the attitudes towards premature and preterm infants at the beginning of your work (examples)?

Institutionalization of Neonatal Care

How did the organization of neonatal care change?
Who initiated the changes?
What resources were mobilized to organize neonatal care?
What sources of information (models of care organization) did you rely on when you organized the neonatal service?
How did it change your work? Your colleagues?
How were the new rules established? Was there resistance (misunderstanding) from the professional community (neonatologists, nurses, obstetricians)?

Current Work and State of the Service

Do you continue to work in the service at present? If no, do you continue to monitor the work of colleagues? If yes, in what status?
What do you see as the main changes in the delivery of neonatal care over the last 40 years? What are the major milestones?
What else could be changed in the organization and work of this service?

Current Professional Work (If Continuing)

How do you see your contribution to the development of neonatology?
What is the most important thing for you in your work? How has it been changing?
What is the most challenging? (including the emotional dimension)

Appendix 2

Guide for a Focus Group with Physicians and Nurses in the Neonatology Service

INTRODUCTION FOR FOCUS GROUP PARTICIPANTS

Good afternoon,

We are researchers from the European University at St. Petersburg, and we invite you to take part in a project on the history of formation and arrangement of neonatal care in St. Petersburg. We wanted to learn about your experience in neonatology, your professional biography and peculiarities of care for newborn patients. As part of the focus group, we would like to focus on the emotional aspects of your profession.

The study is supported by the Associated Professorship on Qualitative Health Research and is conducted in compliance with all ethical standards for social research. Your participation in our project will be anonymous, nor will we identify your place of employment or other personal data or sensitive information. The results of the study will be presented in a summarized form and used for educational, research and scientific purposes only.

If you still have any clarifying questions about the methodology or ethics of the research, you can ask them now or at any stage of the project [researcher contacts]. During the focus group, you may also refuse to answer any of the questions asked and withdraw your consent to participate in the study at any subsequent stage until publication.

We ask your permission to record our conversation for later transcription – Do you consent to be audio-recorded during the focus group?

Introduction of Participants

Age, years of experience, specialty, position, how long they have worked in this particular position

Children and Interaction with Them

What categories / groups of children do you distinguish for yourself? How do you differentiate between them? (*i.e., only by diagnosis – or also by gender, behaviour, other non-medical parameters*). How similar are the needs of different groups of children?

Which groups are the most difficult emotionally to dealand why?

Which groups are satisfying to work with? What does a good day at work mean to you?

Do you interact with the child beyond your job duties and medical manipulations? If so, how, at what times?

To what extent are NICU babies able to communicate, show emotions? Does the behaviour of newborns differ from each other? Can we say that a NICU baby has character and emotions?

Do you find out about the children's health status from other doctors? Do you discuss the condition of children in your free time, or do you discuss the condition of children who are no longer in charge/transferred to another shift? Give an example.

Additional questions/notes for a moderator:

Do you worry about some children more than others? Tell an incident/give an example.

Has your attitude towards children changed during your employment? How much has it been affected by legislative and status changes? (foetus -> child) Developments in technology and medication assistance?

Parents

How much time do you spend interacting with parents (if any at all)? How much (in terms of time) do you interact with them? Why is this seen/not seen as necessary/meaningful?

What groups of parents do you identify? Who is easier to communicate with?

What are the main challenges in communicating with parents?

Emotions

What are the most difficult situations at work? Which ones cause the most concern? What most often triggers your emotions at work? (Communication with co-workers, patients, administration and organizational aspects)

What situations at work cause you the most difficult emotions?

- Regarding children
- Towards parents
- Towards coworkers

How do you deal with the deaths of your patients? Are all deaths experienced in the same way? Why? Give some examples of the deaths you remember the most.

How do you deal with difficult emotions? (fatigue, burnout)

Reflection on Work

To what extent does your work with NICU children impact your personal life?

How do you define professional burnout? How applicable is it to you (self-assessment)? What factors do you think can lead to professional burnout?

What do you see as the meaning of your work? What do you find most important in your work? How has this changed over time?

If you could change your choice now, would you decide to go back to working with neonatal intensive care?

Appendix 3

List of Informants and Description of Interviews

A series of semi-structured interviews with doctors and nurses providing resuscitation and neonatal care and other health practitioners involved in neonatal care (n = 17).

Researchers: A. Novkunskaya, A. Klepikova, A. Minakov

Period of data collection: 2019–2023

Table A3.1 List of informants

No.	*Informant*	*Details*	*Date*	*Interviewers*	*Duration*
1	Doctor RAC	Female, around 70 years old. Intensive care physician, emergency medicine physician. Worked at the RAC since its foundation (1976). Currently work as a consultant	31.01.23	A. Klepikova A. Minakov A. Novkunskaya	2 h. 09 min.
2	Nurse RAC 1	Female, around 65 years old. Intensive care nurse. Worked at the RAC since 1980s.	31.01.23	A. Klepikova A. Minakov	1 h. 07 min.
3	Doctor RAC 2	Female, around 70 years old. Intensive care physician, emergency physician. Worked at the RAC since 1980. One of the developers of the Neonatal Criticality Scale (Formalised information form/blank). Currently work as a consultant.	07.02.23	A. Klepikova A. Minakov A. Novkunskaya	1 h. 18 min.
4	Head of one of the first NICUs in Russia	Male, more than 75 years old. Paediatrician, intensive care physician. Former head of the neonatal intensive care unit. One of the founders of neonatal resuscitation in the region. Currently in retirement.	28.02.23	A. Minakov A. Novkunskaya	1 h. 16 min.
5	Head of NICU at a large surgical hospital	Female, around 50 years old. Emergency room physician. Deputy chief physician in a paediatric hospital. Former head of the neonatal intensive care unit.	20.03.23	A. Klepikova A. Novkunskaya	46 min.
6	Head of neonatal unit of the paediatrician hospital	Female, around 70 years old. Neonatologist. Head of neonatal unit of paediatric hospital.	03.05.23	A. Novkunskaya	58 min
7	Head of the intensive care unit paediatrician hospital	Male, around 40 years old. Formerly a physician in the neonatal intensive care unit. Currently works as the head of the intensive care unit for older children (not newborns).	19.04.23	A. Novkunskaya	1 h. 43 min.

8	Head of the neonatal department of the maternity hospital	Male, around 35 years old. Resuscitation physician with experience in NICU departments of different regions. Currently works as a deputy chief physician for neonatology at a private hospital.	23.05.23	A. Minakov A. Novkunskaya	2 h. 53 min.
9	Doctor working in the palliative paediatric service	Male, around 55 years old. Resuscitation physician. Has experience in a high administrative position of a regional hospital (another region)	06.06.23	A. Novkunskaya	59 min.
10	Head of neonatal unit of the paediatrician hospital	Female, around 60 years old. Neonatologist. Former emergency physician. Head of neonatal unit of paediatric hospital.	13.09.23	A. Klepikova A. Minakov A. Novkunskaya	1 h. 57 min.
11	The deputy chief physician for administrative and expert work	Female, around 55 years old. Former paediatrician.	17.10.23	A. Novkunskaya	27 min.
12	Doctor RAC (mobile team)	Female, around 40 years old. Intensive care physician. Worked in several intensive care departments, including a major federal centre. Currently works in mobile RAC team.	01.03.20	A. Minakov	51 min.
13	Intensive care physician of maternity hospital	Female, around 40 years old. Intensive care physician, neonatologist. Worked in several maternity hospitals and paediatric hospitals. Currently works as a physician in NICU of a maternity hospital.	10.11.21	A. Minakov	1 h. 45 min.
14	Intensive care physician of maternity hospital	Female, around 30 years old. Intensive care physician, neonatologist. Has working experience in only one major maternity hospital after residency. Currently works as a physician in NICU of a maternity hospital.	29.11.21	A. Minakov	49 min.

(*Continued*)

Table A3.1 (Continued)

No.	*Informant*	*Details*	*Date*	*Interviewers*	*Duration*
15	Head of the department of catamnesis	Female, around 40 years old. Paediatrician. Has working experience in several paediatric hospitals. Currently works as a head of the department of catamnesis in one of the paediatric hospitals.	02.03.22	A. Minakov	31 min.
16	Intensive care physician of maternity hospital, part-time RAC mobile team doctor	Female, around 30 years old. Intensive care physician, neonatologist. Has working experience in several maternity hospitals. Currently works as a physician in NICU of a maternity hospital and as a part-time RAC mobile team doctor.	18.01.22	A. Minakov	34 min.
17	Doctor RAC (mobile team)	Female, around 30 years old. Intensive care physician, neonatologist. Worked in neonatal care unit in different regions. Currently works as a RAC mobile team doctor.	16.11.19	A. Minakov	52 min.

Appendix 4

List of Observations

This dataset includes details on ethnographic observations conducted within the hospitals and RAC in 2019–2023. The goals were to study communications within and between medical employees and different departments of neonatal care system, as well as interactions with patients and their parents. The dataset includes 21 diverse locations (medical units). Self-observation by Minakov A. in the course of his own work as a transport intensive care team physician – 33 on-call visits over a three-year period (92 pages of diary entries). Participant observation of the work of the medical staff of the transport intensive care service, maternity hospitals and the intensive care unit of the paediatric hospital (75 pages of diary entries).

Researchers: A. Novkunskaya, A. Klepikova, A.Minakov

Table A4.1 List of observations

	Researcher	Date	Location	Number of Pages in Field Diary
1	A. Minakov	11.12.2019	Maternity hospital P, paediatric hospital A	3
2	A. Minakov	13.12.2019	Paediatric hospital A, maternity hospital P, maternity hospital Q	6
3	A. Minakov	17.12.2019	Paediatric hospital A, RAC	1
4	A. Minakov	27.12.2019	Paediatric hospital A, RAC, maternity hospital R	4
5	A. Minakov	29.11.2019	Paediatric hospital A, RAC, maternity hospital R	2
6	A. Minakov	29.12.2019	Paediatric hospital A, maternity hospital R, maternity hospital I, multispecialty hospital B.	4
7	A. Minakov	01.01.2020	Maternity hospital R, maternity hospital M	6
8	A. Minakov	03.01.2020	Paediatric hospital B, maternity hospital P	4
9	A. Minakov	06.01.2020	Multispecialty hospital P, maternity hospital A, federal maternity hospital	5
10	A. Minakov	14.01.2020	Multispecialty hospital B, maternity hospital F, maternity hospital P	4
11	A. Minakov	17.01.2020	Maternity hospital F, maternity hospital R	3
12	A. Minakov A. Klepikova	20.01.2020	Multispecialty hospital B, maternity hospital P	16
13	A. Minakov	22.01.2020	Multispecialty hospital B, paediatric hospital C	4
14	A. Minakov	24.01.2020	Federal maternity hospital	5
15	A. Minakov	27.01.2020	Maternity hospital J, maternity hospital R	
16	A. Minakov	30.01.2020	Multispecialty hospital P	1
17	A. Minakov	03.02.2020	Maternity hospital R, Maternity hospital F	3
18	A. Minakov	15.02.2023 17.02.2023	Maternity hospital P	3
19	A. Minakov	26.02.2020	Multispecialty hospital P, paediatric hospital A	3
20	A. Minakov	08.03.2020 13.03.2020 17.03.2020	Private maternity clinic 2, maternity hospital M, perinatal centre O	5
21	A. Minakov	02.03.2020	Private maternity clinic 1, maternity hospital Q	3

(*Continued*)

Table A4.1 (Continued)

	Researcher	*Date*	*Location*	*Number of pages in Field Diary*
22	A. Minakov	21.08.2020, 26.08.2020 28.08.2020	Maternity hospital I, maternity hospital J, private maternity clinic 2	4
23	A. Minakov	09.09.2020	Multispecialty hospital P	
24	A. Minakov	09.10.2020	Maternity hospital I, maternity hospital P, paediatric hospital D	7
25	A. Minakov	12.10.2020	Maternity hospital A, maternity hospital J	3
26	A. Minakov	16.10.2020	Maternity hospital R, paediatric hospital A	2
27	A. Minakov	06.11.2020	Maternity hospital P	2
28	A. Minakov	26.03.2020	Perinatal centre P	2
29	A. Minakov	07.04.2021	Maternity hospital I	3
30	A. Novkunskaya	05.06.2023	Paediatric hospital A, RAC, neonatal unit of paediatric hospital, maternity hospital J, privet maternity clinic 2	6
31	A. Klepikova	13.06.2023	Paediatric hospital A, RAC, maternity hospital R	9
32	A. Klepikova	11.07.2023	Paediatric hospital A, RAC, maternity hospital R	14
33	A. Novkunskaya	30.07.2023	Paediatric hospital A, RAC, neonatal unit of paediatric hospital, maternity hospital I, paediatric hospital B, maternity hospital P	13
34	A. Novkunskaya	22.11.2023	Paediatric hospital A conference	4
35	A. Klepikova	10.01.2020	Paediatric hospital A, RAC, maternity hospital A.	13
		In total:	21 diverse locations	167 pages

Appendix 5

List and Description of Focus Groups

RESEARCHERS: A. NOVKUNSKAYA, A. KLEPIKOVA AND A. MINAKOV

Table A5.1 List of Focus-groups

Group	*Participants*	*Researchers*	*Duration*	*Location*
Reanimatologists-neonatologists, working in RAC	1. Male, working experience of 15 years. 2. Male, working experience of 45 years. 3. Female, working experience of 23 years, 4. Female, working experience of 23 years,	A. Klepikova A. Novkunskaya	09.40–11.00	RAC
Neonatologists working in different maternity hospitals in the City	1. Female, working experience of 6 years. 2. Female, working experience of 6 years. 3. Female, working experience of 19 years. 4. Female, working experience of 42 years. 5. Female, working experience of 18 years. 6. Female, working experience of 22 years.	A. Klepikova A. Novkunskaya A. Minakov	17.50–19.20	European University at St.Petersburg
Reanimatologists, working in NICU of a paediatric hospital	1. Male, working experience of 29 years. 2. Female, working experience of 20 years. 3. Male, working experience of 2 years. 4. Male, working experience of 7 years. 5. Female, working experience of 20 years. 6. Male, working experience of 6 years. 7. Male, working experience of 29 years 8. Male, working experience of 15 years	A. Klepikova A. Novkunskaya A. Minakov	09.55–11.05	RAC
Neonatologists, working in a neonatal unit of a paediatric hospital	1. Female, working experience of 13 years, 2. Female, working experience of 17 years, 3. Female, working experience of 4 years, 4. Female, working experience of 4 years	A. Klepikova A. Novkunskaya A. Minakov	16.30–17.30	European University at St.Petersburg

Nurses of neonatal units in Maternity hospitals and RAC	1. Female, working experience of 10 years (midwifery education, last 6 years work as a head nurse of a paediatric department in Perinatal centre). 2. Female, working experience about 8 years (midwifery education, Nurse of NICU, RAC nurse) 3. Male, working experience of 15 years (nurse of NICU, head nurse, nurse RAC) 4. Female, working experience of 7 years—(nurse of NICU perinatal centre). 5. Female, working experience 14 years. (midwife education, nurse of NICU, Head nurse, nurse RAC)	A. Klepikova, A. Novkunskaya,	15.00–16.35	European University at St.Petersburg
Nurses, working in a NICU of a paediatric hospital	1. Female, working experience of 22 years 2. Male, working experience of 4 years 3. Female, working experience of 23 years 4. Female, working experience of 8 years 5. Female, working experience of 23 years 6. Female, working experience of 13 years	A. Klepikova, A. Novkunskaya,	09.50–10.30	Peadiatric hospital **A** conference hall
Total participants:	33 practitioners			

Appendix 6

List of Archival Documents

Documents relevant to the history of neonatal service in the study region and neonatal care in Russia (scanned copies):

1. Temporary regulations on the neonatology mobile team, agreed by the chief paediatrician, chief paediatric surgeon, chief physician of the ambulance station, 1976 (two pages).
2. Temporary regulations on the work of twentieth specialised paediatric emergency medical station, agreed by the chief paediatrician, chief paediatric surgeon, chief physician of the emergency medical station, 1977 (four pages).
3. Order 888 of the Main Health Department of the City Executive Committee dated 30.07.1977 on the organisation of Children's Hospital A (three pages).
4. Main Health Department of the Executive Committee of the Lensovet. Order No. 438 of 05.05.1980 on the establishment of a resuscitation and consultation centre for children's hospitals (two pages).
5. Attachment to Order No. 438 of 05.05.1980 on the establishment of a resuscitation and consultation centre for children's hospitals (three pages).
6. Instructions for the use of FIB-014 formalised information form of an insert in the medical history of a newborn in a maternity hospital, 1986 (four pages).
7. Regulations on the Scientific and Practical Association for Pediatric Resuscitation Care, approved by the Head of the Main Health Department of the Executive Committee of the Lensoviet Executive Committee (1980s) (two pages).

8. Formalised information form (FIB-016) of the Laboratory of Automated Management Systems in Pediatrics of the Leningrad Main Health Department and the Leningrad Pediatric University (By V. P. Antonova, M. D. Matyushkina, E. Z. Proskurova Laboratory of Pediatric Informatics 1990) (two pages).

References

Abu-Lughod, L. (2016). *Veiled sentiments: Honor and poetry in a Bedouin society*. California: University of California Press.

Acocella, I. (2011). The focus groups in social research: Advantages and disadvantages. *Quality & Quantity*, 46(4), 1125–1136.

Ahmed, S. (2013). *The cultural politics of emotion*. New York: Routledge.

Anspach, R. R. (1993). *Deciding who lives: Fateful choices in the intensive-care nursery*. California: University of California Press.

Antonov, A. G., Burov, A. A., Volodin, N. N., Gorev, V. V., Degtyarev, D. N., Degtyareva, M. V., . . . & Filippov, O. S. (2020). Resuscitation and stabilization of newborn babies in the delivery room. Methodological letter/edited by Prof. EN Baibarina. M., 2020. Neonatology: News. Opinions. *Training*, 8(27), 34–52. (in Russian).

Avdeeva, A. (2020). Natural parenting in contemporary Russia: When 'nature' meets kinship. Doctoral Dissertation. Helsinki. Publications of the Faculty of Arts Doctoral Programme in Gender, Culture and Society, SKY.

Baiburin, A. K. (2017). *Soviet passport: History - structure - practices*. St.Petersburg: Publishing house of the European University in St. Petersburg. (in Russian).

Baiburin, A. K. (1993). Ritual in traditional culture. Structural and Semantic Analysis of Eastern Slavic Rites. *SPb: Science*, 237. (in Russian).

Beatty, A. (2014). Anthropology and emotion. *Journal of the Royal Anthropological Institute*, 20(3), 545–563.

Becker, H. S. (1963). *Outsiders. Studies in the sociology of deviance*. New York: The Free Press of Glencoe.

Becker, H. S., Geer, B., Hughes, E. C., & Strauss, A. L. (1961). *Boys in white: Student culture in medical school*. Chicago: University of Chicago Press.

Berg, M. (1996). Practices of reading and writing: The constitutive role of the patient record in medical work. *Sociology of Health & Illness*, 18(4), 499–524.

Berg, M., & Bowker, G. (1997). The multiple bodies of the medical record: Toward a sociology of an artifact. *Sociological Quarterly*, 38(3), 513–537.

Bill No. 510787-8 "On Amending Article 56 of the Federal Law 'On the Fundamentals of Health Protection of Citizens in the Russian Federation'" (2023). Available at: https://sozd.duma.gov.ru/bill/510787-8 (access date 09.01.2024).

Borozdina, E., Elnitckii, E., & Khodorenko, D. (2022). Prove of harm: Patient experiences and medical standards in court decisions. *The Journal of Social Policy Studies*, 20(2), 199–214. https://doi.org/10.17323/727-0634-2022-20-2-199-214 (in Russian).

Borozdina, E. (2018). Introducing 'natural' childbirth in Russian hospitals. Midwives' institutional work. *Health, technologies, and politics in post-Soviet settings: Navigating uncertainties*, (pp. 145–171). New York: Palgrave Macmillan US.

Borozdina, E. (2023). Evidence-based medicine and physicians' institutional agency in Russian clinical settings. *Critical Public Health*, 33, 1–12.

Borozdina, E., & Novkunskaya, A. (2022). Patient-centered care in Russian maternity hospitals: Introducing a new approach through professionals' agency. *Health*, 26(2), 200–220.

Breen, Lauren, J. (2007). The researcher 'in the middle': Negotiating the insider/outsider dichotomy. *The Australian Community Psychologist,* 19(1), 163–174.

C. T. E. Jr. (1981). L'Hôpital des Enfants-Malades, the world's first children's hospital, founded in Paris in 1802. *Pediatrics*, 67(5), 670–670.

Carroll, A. E., & Buddenbaum, J. L. (2013). High and low-risk specialties experience with the US medical malpractice system. *BMC Health Services Research*, 13, 1–7.

Chernova, J. V. (2013). Gender analysis of family policy in modern Russia: Features and trends [Gendernyj analiz semejnoj politiki v sovremennoj Rossii: osobennosti i tendencii.]. (in Russian)

Clemente, I. (2015). *Uncertain futures communication and culture in childhood cancer treatment.* New Jersey: Wiley-Blackwell.

Conrad, P. (1992). Medicalization and social control. *Annual Review of Sociology*, 18, 209–232.

Cook, L. J. (2011). Russia's Wellfare Regime: The shift toward statism, in M. Jäppinen, M. Kulmala, & A. Saarinen (Eds.), *Gazing at welfare, gender and agency in post-socialist Countries* (pp.14–37). Cambridge: Cambridge Scholars Publishing.

Cook, L. J. (2015). Constraints on universal health care in the Russian Federation: Inequality, informality and the failures of mandatory health insurance reforms. *Journal of Self-Governance and Management Economics*, 3(4), 37–60.

Csordas, T. J. (2002). Somatic modes of attention, in Csordas, T. J. *Body/meaning/healing* (pp. 241–259). New York: Palgrave Macmillan US.

Davis-Floyd, R. (2001). The technocratic, humanistic, and holistic paradigms of childbirth. *International Journal of Gynecology & Obstetrics*, 75, S5–S23.

Davis-Floyd, Robbie. (2004). *Birth as an American rite of passage: With a new preface.* California: University of California Press.

De Vries, Raymond, Benoit, C., Van Teijlingen, E., & Wrede, S. (2002). *Birth by design: Pregnancy, maternity care and midwifery in North America and Europe.* New York: Routledge.

Decree 888 of 30.06.1977 On the organization of work of children's city hospital No. 1(in Russian)

Decree of the Government of the Russian Federation No. 1734-r of 04.12.07 (in Russian)

Decree of the Government of the Russian Federation No. 2302-r of 09.12.13 (in Russian)

Decree of the Ministry of Health and Social Development of the Russian Federation of December 27, 2011 N 1687n "On medical criteria for birth, the form of the birth document and the procedure for its issuance" (as amended and supplemented). (in Russian)

Decree of the Ministry of Health of the Russian Federation of 04.12.1992. (in Russian)

Decree of the Ministry of Health of the Russian Federation of 20.10.2020 N 1130n "On Approval of the Procedure for the provision of medical care in the profile "obstetrics and gynecology" (in Russian)

Decree of the Ministry of Health of the Russian Federation of August 19, 2020 N 869n "On approval of general requirements for the organization of visits to the patient by relatives and other family members or legal representatives of the patient in a medical organization, including in its structural subdivisions designed for intensive care and resuscitation measures, when providing medical care in inpatient settings" (in Russian).

Decree of the Ministry of Health of the Russian Federation of November 15, 2012, No. 921n "On Approval of the Procedure for the Provision of Medical Care in the Profile of Neonatology". (in Russian)

Decree of the Ministry of Health of the USSR dated November 4, 1987 N 1178 "On making additions to the nomenclature of medical specialties and medical positions". (in Russian)

Delektorsky, N. I. (1910). Mortality of children Abroad, in Russia and in Tomsk and "A Drop of Milk"[Smertnost' detej za granicej, v Rossii i v Tomske i «Kaplya Moloka]. Tomsk: Tipography of the provincial administration. - 24 c. (in Russian).

Deligianni, M., Voultsos, P., Tzitiridou-Chatzopoulou, M. K., Drosou-Agakidou, V., & Tarlatzis, V. (2023). Moral distress among neonatologists working in neonatal intensive care units in Greece: A qualitative study. *BMC Pediatrics*, 23(1), 114.

Di Renzo, G. C. (2020). Expert report on the Elina Sushkevich case. *Акушерство, г инекология и репродукция*, 14(6), 710–714.

Dingwall, R., & Murray, T. (1983). Categorization in accident departments: 'Good' patients, 'bad' patients and 'children'. *Sociology of Health & Illness*, 5(2), 127–148.

Douglas, M. (2003). *Purity and danger: An analysis of concepts of pollution and taboo.*New York: Routledge.

Durkheim, E. (1995|1912). *The elementary forms of religious life*. New York: Free Press.

Dwyer, Sonya Corbin, & Buckle, J. L. (2009). The space between: On being an insider-outsider in qualitative research. *International Journal of Qualitative Methods,* 8(1), 54–63.

Edelman Lauren, Suchman Mark. (1997). The Legal Environments of Organizations. Annual.

Edwards, Paul. (2002). Infrastructure and Modernity: Scales of Force. Time, and Social Organization in the History of Sociotechnical Systems. Modernity and Technology. Cambridge, MA: MIT Press, pp. 185–225.

Ekman, P. (1980). *Face of man: Universal expression in a New Guinea village.* New York: Garland.

Ekman, P. (1984). Expression and the nature of emotion, in K. Scherer, & P. Ekman (Eds.), *Approaches to emotion* (pp. 319–343). Hillsdale, New Jersey: Erlbaum.

Fainzang, S. (2007). Anthropology and medicine: Empathy, experience and knowledge. *Wiener ethnomedizinische Reihe*, 4, 1–20.

Featherstone, M. (2020). Towards a bureaucracy of the body. *New formations*, 100(100–101), 97–113.

Federal Law of March 4, 2022 No. 32-FZ "On Amendments to the Criminal Code of the Russian Federation and Articles 31 and 151 of the Criminal Procedure Code of the Russian Federation". Available at the link: https://www.consultant.ru/document/cons_doc_LAW_410887/ (in Russian) (access date 10.01.2024).

Ferguson, C. A. (1964). Baby talk in six languages. *American Anthropologist*, 66(6), 103–114.

Ferrie, J., & Wiseman, P. (2019). 'Running out of time': Exploring the concept of waiting for people with Motor Neurone Disease. *Time & Society*, 28(2), 521–542.

Field, M. G. (1957). *Doctor and patient in Soviet Russia.* Cambridge: Harvard University Press.

Field, M. G. (1988). The position of the Soviet physician: The bureaucratic professional. *The Milbank Quarterly*, 66(2), 182–201.

Fitzpatrick, S. (2005). *Tear off the masks!* Princeton: Princeton University Press.

Flick, U. (2009). *An introduction to qualitative research* (4th ed.). London: SAGE Publications Ltd.

Foucault, M. (1988). Technologies of the self. In Martin L.H., Gutman H. and Hutton P.H. (Eds.), Technologies of the Self: A Seminar with Michel Foucault. (pp. 16-49). Amherst: The University of Massachusetts Press.

Freidson, E. (1988). *Profession of medicine: A study of the sociology of applied knowledge.* Chicago: University of Chicago Press.

Freidson, E. (2001). *Professionalism, the third logic: On the practice of knowledge.* Chicago: University of Chicago press.

Geertz, C. (2008). Thick description: Toward an interpretive theory of culture, in Oakes, T., & Price, P. L. (Eds.), *The cultural geography reader* (pp. 41–51). New York: Routledge.

Goffman, E. (1961). *Asylums: Essays on the Social Situation of Mental Patients and Other Inmates.* New York: Anchor books.

Goffman, E. (1963). *Stigma: Notes on the management of spoiled identity.* Englewood Cliffs: Prentice-Hall.

Goffman, E. (1956). *The presentation of self in everyday life.* Edinburgh: University of Edinburgh.

Goffman, E. (1959). The moral career of the mental patient. *Psychiatry*, 22(2), 123–142.

Goffman, E. (1974). Frame analysis: An essay on the organization of experience. Cambridge: Harvard University Press.

Gonzalez, R. M., & Gilleskie, D. (2017). Infant mortality rate as a measure of a country's health: A robust method to improve reliability and comparability. *Demography*, 54(2), 701–720.

Goold, I., & Herring, J. (2018). *Great debates in medical law and ethics*. London: Bloomsbury Publishing.

Gorbachev, V. I., Netesin, E. S., Kozlov, A. I., Sumin, S. A., & Gorbacheva, S. M. (2020). Analytical review on criminal cases against anesthesiologists-anesthesiolo gists-resuscitators over the last five years. *Bulletin of Intensive Care named after AI Saltanov*, 1, 19–24. (in Russian).

Gorelova, L. E., & Shelkova, V. N. From the fight against puerperal infections to overcoming infant mortality, from obstetrics to pediatrics. Byulleten' Nacional'nogo nauchno-issledovatel'skogo instituta obshchestvennogo zdorov'ya imeni N.A. Semashko [Bulletin of Semashko National Research Institute of Public Health]. 2022. No. 1–2. P. 118–123 (in Russian). DOI: 10.25742/NRIPH.2022.01.013.

Gras, T. (2022). Alexandre lion: The forgotten inventor of incubator shows. *Pediatrics*, 150(3). https://doi.org/10.1542/peds.2021-054576.

Heart to Heart. Global cardiac care. About us: https://www.heart-2-heart.org/about-us (accessed 18.05.2023).

Hochschild, A. R. (1979). Emotion work, feeling rules, and social structure. *American Journal of Sociology*, 85(3), 551–575.

Hochschild, A. (1983). *The managed heart*. Berkeley: University of California.

Hughes, T P. (1987). The evolution of large technological systems in the social construction of technological systems: New Directions in the Sociology and History of Technology. Cambridge, MA: MIT Press.

Hull, M. S. (2008). Ruled by records: The expropriation of land and the misappropriation of lists in Islamabad. *American Ethnologist*, 35(4), 501–518. https://doi.org/10.1111/j.1548-1425.2008.00095.x.

Humphrey, Caroline. (2007). Insider-outsider: Activating the hyphen. *Action Research,* 5(1), 11–26.

Illich, I. (1976). *Medical nemesis: The expropriation of health*. New York: Pantheon Books.

Illouz, E. (2008). *Saving the modern soul: Therapy, emotions, and the culture of self-help*. California: University of California Press.

Investigative Committee of the Russian Federation. (2019). A criminal case has been opened over the murder of a newborn baby in a maternity hospital in the Kaliningrad region. Available at: https://sledcom.ru/news/item/1369103 (in Russian) (Accessed 09.01.2024).

Ivanov, V. M. (1911). Infant mortality and the importance of "Drop of Milk" in the fight against it [Detskaya smertnost' i znachenie «Kapli Moloka» v bor'be s neyu.]. Novocherkassk: Printing House "Donskoy Pechatnik. (in Russian).

Jena, A. B., Seabury, S., Lakdawalla, D., & Chandra, A. (2011). Malpractice risk according to physician specialty. *New England Journal of Medicine*, 365(7), 629–636.

Kerstetter, Katie. (2012). Insider, outsider, or somewhere between: The impact of researchers' identitieson the community-based research process. *Journal of Rural Social Sciences*, 27(2), 7.

Khazanov, A. I. (1973). Nursing of premature infants [Vyhazhivanie nedonoshennyh detej]. - L.: Medicine. Leningr. department. - 206 c (in Russian).

Kirmayer, L. J., & Robbins, J. M. (1996). Patients who somatize in primary care: A longitudinal study of cognitive and social characteristics. *Psychological Medicine*, 26(5), 937–951.

Kleinman, A. (2020). Concepts and a model for the comparison of medical systems as cultural systems, in Currer C., Stacey M. (Eds.), *Concepts of health, illness and disease* (pp. 27–47). New York: Routledge.

Klepikova, A. A., & Utekhin, I. V. (2010). A child with "developmental disabilities": The experience of frame analysis. *Anthropological Forum*, 12, 1–68. (In Russian).

Klepikova, A. (2017). Social construction of mental disabilities in Russian residential care institutions. *Public Health Panorama*, 3(1), 22–30.

Klepikova, A. (2019). Curing disability in contemporary Russia: Rehabilitation practices and the placebo effect. *Ethnologia Polona*, 40, 49–65.

Klepikova, A., Altukhova, A., & Mokhov, S. (2023). On the results of the study "Communication between doctors, volunteers and patients with ALS: Problems and ways to solve them", report at the VIII Annual Conference on ALS of the Foundation "Live Now", (Moscow, May 18–19, 2023). (in Russian).

Korobeev, A. I., & Shirshov, A. A. (2020). Kriterii zhivorozhdeniya pri opredelenii zhizni kak obyekta ugolovno—pravovoy okhrany [Criteria of live birth in determining life as an object of criminal legal protection]. *Lex Russica*, (5 (162)), 64–72. (in Russian).

Kvale, S. (2003). *Research interview*. Moscow: Sense. (In Russian).

Lakoff, G. (1987). *Women, fire and dangerous things*. Chicago: University of Chicago Press.

Latour, B., & Woolgar, S. (2013). *Laboratory life: The construction of scientific facts*. Princeton: Princeton university press.

Lavrov, V. (1983). The house of motherhood. *Agitator's Notebook*, 13, 46–59. (in Russian).

Leavitt, J. (1996). Meaning and feeling in the anthropology of emotions. *American Ethnologist*, 23(3), 514–539.

Leikin, N. A. (1907). In his memoirs and correspondence. St. Petersburg: R. Golike and A. Villorg.(in Russian).

Lemert, E. M. (1951). *Social pathology; A systematic approach to the theory of sociopathic behavior*. New York: McGraw-Hill Book Company.

Levy, R. (1982). On the nature and functions of the emotions: An anthropological perspective. *Information sur les Sciences Sociales Paris*, 21(4–5), 511–528.

Lindholm, C. (2005). An anthropology of emotion, in *Casey, C., & Edgerton, R. B. (Eds.), A companion to psychological anthropology: Modernity and psychocultural change* (pp. 30–47). Blackwell companions to anthropology (4) Malden, MA: Blackwell.

Litvina, D. (2022). Reproductive losses in the context of institutional interaction: Practices, spaces and trajectories of care. *The Journal of Social Policy Studies*, 20(2), 215–228. (In Russian).

Litvina, D., Novkunskaya, A., & Temkina, A. (2019). Multiple vulnerabilities in medical settings: Invisible suffering of doctors. *Societies*, 10(1), 5.

Loginov, A. V., & Zainulina, M. S. (2017). The golden pages in the Russian history of obstetrics: From the times of Ekaterine to the present. *Obstetrics, Gynecology and Reproduction*, 11(2), 69–74. (in Russian).

Lorber, Judith. (1975). Good patients and problem patients: Conformity and deviance in a general hospital. *Journal of Health and Social Behavior*, 16(2), 213–225.

Lupton, D. (2012). *Medicine as culture: Illness, disease and the body*. London: Sage.

Lutz, C. (1986). Emotion, thought, and estrangement: Emotion as a cultural category. *Cultural Anthropology*, 1(3), 287–309.

Lutz, C. A. (2011). Unnatural emotions: Everyday sentiments on a Micronesian atoll and their challenge to Western theory. Chicago: University of Chicago Press.

Lutz, C., & White, G. M. (1986). The anthropology of emotions. *Annual Review of Anthropology*, 15(1), 405–436.

Lyubimenko, V. A., Pankratov, L. G., & Mostovoy, A. V. (2005). The use of kurosurf in neonatology [Primenenie Kurosurfa v neonatologii]. *Lechaschi Vrach Journal*, 10, 89–91. (in Russian).

Malinowski, B. (2013|1922). *Argonauts of the western Pacific: An account of native enterprise and adventure in the archipelagoes of Melanesian New Guinea [1922/1994]*. New York: Routledge.

Mansurov, V. A., & Yurchenko, O. V. (2004). Perspectives of professionalization of Russian doctors in a reforming society. *Russia Reforming*, 4, 61–79. (in Russian).

Marshall, D. A. (2002). Behavior, belonging, and belief: A theory of ritual practice. *Sociological Theory*, 20(3), 360–380.

Matveev, I., & Novkunskaya, A. (2022). Welfare restructuring in Russia since 2012: National trends and evidence from the regions. *Europe-Asia Studies*, 74(1), 50–71.

Mikhel' D. V. (2009). Medikalizatsiya obshchestva: teoriya, istoriya, mikropolitika [Medicalization of Society: Theory, History and Micropolitics]. *Zhurnal issledovaniy sotsial'noy politiki [The Journal of Social Policy Studies]*, 7(4), 293–294.

Mikhel' D. V. (2011). Medikalizatsiya kak sotsial'nyy fenomen [Medicalization as a Social Phenomenon]. Vestnik Saratovskogo gosudarstvennogo tekhnicheskogo universiteta [Bulletin of the Saratov State Technical University], 4(2 (60)), 256–263.

Mitsyuk, N. A., & Pokusaeva, V. N. (2016). Pregnancy management in pre-revolutionary Russia: From traditional practices to medical knowledge [Vedenie beremennosti v dorevolyucionnoj Rossii: ot tradicionnyh praktik k medicinskomu znaniyu]. *Bulletin of Smolensk State Medical Academy*, 15(2), 85–93. (in Russian).

Mitsyuk, N. A., & Pushkareva, N. L. (2021). The development of the system of clinical obstetrics in Russia (from the late eighteenth to the early twentieth century) [Formirovanie sistemy klinichkskogo rodovspomozheniya v Rossii (konec XVIII-nachalo XX V.)]. *History of Medicine*, 7(2), 153–160. (in Russian).

Mitsyuk, N. A., Belova, A. V., & Pushkareva, N. L. (2021). Sourse potential of the founds on maternity hospitals and wards in pre-revolutionary Russia: Second half of the 18th-early 20th century [Istochnikovedcheskij potencial fondov rodil'nyh domov i otdelenij v dorevolyucionnoj Rossii. Vtoraya polovina XVIII-nachalo XXv]. *Vestnik archivista*, 4, 1009–1022. (in Russian).

Mitsyuk, N. A., Pushkareva, N. L., & Belova, A. V. (2022). Organization of the space of the first maternity clinics in Russia (XVIII-begining of the XX centuries) [Organizaciya prostranstva pervyh rodil'nyh klinik v Rossii (XIX-nachalo XX vv.)]. *Bylye Gody*, 17(2), 621–670. (in Russian).

Mitsyuk, N. A., & Pushkareva, N. L. Domashnie rody v rossiiskikh dvorianskikh sem'iakh (konets XIX – nachalo XX v.) [Home Childbirth in Russian Noble Families (Late 19th – Early 20th Centuries)] *Ethnographic Review*, 5, 167–183. (in Russian).

Mokhov, S., & Novkunskaya, A. A. (2021). Infrastructural breaks on the road from birth to death in contemporary Russia. *Religions*, 12(12), 1115.

Mol, A. (2002). *The body multiple: Ontology in medical practice*. Durham: Duke University Press.

Moreira, T., & Palladino, P. (2005). Between truth and hope: On Parkinson's disease, neurotransplantation and the production of the 'self'. *History of the Human Sciences*, 18(3), 55–82.

Murphy, R. F. (1987). *The body silent*. New York: Henry Holt.

Mustafina-Bredikhina, D. M. (2017). Iatrogenic crimes as a new trend in modern society. Neonatology: News. Opinions. *Training*, 4(18), 168–170. (in Russian).

Najman, J. M., Klein, D., & Munro, C. (1982). Patient characteristics negatively stereotyped by doctors. *Social Science & Medicine*, 16(20), 1781–1789.

Nápoles-Springer, A. M., Santoyo, J., Houston, K., Pérez-Stable, E. J., & Stewart, A. L. (2005). Patients' perceptions of cultural factors affecting the quality of their medical encounters. *Health Expectations*, 8(1), 4–17.

Novikov, B. N. (2010). Midwifery service of Saint-Petersburg: Yesterday, today, tomorrow. *Journal of Obstetrics and Women's Diseases*, LIX (1), 11–17. (in Russian).

Novkunskaya, A. (2020). *Professional agency and institutional change: Case of maternity services in small-town Russia*. Helsinki: University of Helsinki.

Novkunskaya, A., Litvina, D., & Temkina, A. (2021). "Sociologists in white": Constructing a professional position in the medical field. *Laboratorium: A Journal of Social Research*, 3, 57–87. (In Russian).

Ortner, S. B. (2016). Dark anthropology and its others: Theory since the eighties. *HAU: Journal of Ethnographic Theory*, 6(1), 47–73.

Paneyakh, E. (2014). Faking performances together: Systems of performance evaluation in Russian enforcement agencies and production of bias and privilege. *Post-Soviet Affairs*, 30(2–3), 115–136.

Parsons, T. (1951a). Illness and the role of the physician: A sociological perspective. *American Journal of Orthopsychiatry*, 21(3), 452–460.

Parsons, T. (1951b). *The social system*. Glencoe, IL: The Free Press.

Passport of the national project "Health Care" (approved by the Presidium of the Presidential Council for Strategic Development and National Projects, Minutes of December 24, 2018 N 16): https://base.garant.ru/72185920/ (in Russian).

Pavlova, V. N., & Zelentsova, V. L. (2020). The formation of native neonatology [K istorii razvitiya otechestvennoj neonatologii].In Collection of articles" V International (75 All-Russian) scientific-practical conference "Actual issues of modern medical science and health care". 2020.№ 2. Federal State Budgetary Educational Institution of Higher Education "Ural State Medical University" of the Ministry of Health of the Russian Federation. (in Russian).

Petersen, A., Seear, K., & Munsie, M. (2014). Therapeutic journeys: The hopeful travails of stem cell tourists. *Sociology of Health & Illness*, 36(5), 670–685.

Powdermaker, H. (1966). *Stranger and friend: The way of an anthropologist* (No. 410). New York: WW Norton & Company.

Pushkareva, N. L., & Mitsyuk, N. A., (2017). The origins of medicalization: The basis of Russian social policy in the field of reproductive health (1760–1860). *Journal of Social Policy Studies*, 15(4), 515–530. (in Russian).

Radbill, S. X. (1955). A history of children's hospitals. *AMA American Journal of Diseases of Children*, 90(4), 411–416.

Reddy, W. M. (1997). Against constructionism: The historical ethnography of emotions. *Current Anthropology*, 38(3), 327–351.

Reddy, W. M. (2001). *The navigation of feeling: A framework for the history of emotions*. Cambridge: Cambridge University Press.

Reddy, W. M. (2008). Emotional styles and modern forms of life. Sexualized brains: Scientific modeling of emotional intelligence from a cultural perspective, (pp. 81–100). Cambridge, MA: MIT Press.

Report St. Petersburg City Executive Sanitary Commission for 1901. 1901, p. 75 (in Russian).

Resolution of the State Statistics Committee of Russia dated 04.12.1992 No. 190 (in Russian).

Ridgeway, C. L. (2009). Framed before we know it: How gender shapes social relations. *Gender & Society*, 23(2), 145–160.

Ries, N. (1997). *Russian talk: Culture and conversation during perestroika*. New York: Cornell University Press.

Rispoli, Giulia. (2015). The path of cybernetics in the Soviet Union: From rejection to celebration in the service of communism. *Paradigmi: rivista di critica filosofica*, XXXIII(3), 149–162.

Rivkin-Fish, M. (2010). Pronatalism, gender politics, and the renewal of family support in Russia: Toward a feminist anthropology of "maternity capital". *Slavic review*, 69(3), 701–724.

Robinson, I., & Hunter, M. (1998). *Motor neurone disease*. London: Psychology Press.

Rodriguez, N. M., & Ryave, A. (2002). *Systematic self-observation: A method for researching the hidden and elusive features of everyday social life* (Vol. 49). London: Sage.

Rodziewicz, T. L., & Hipskind, J. E. (2020). *Medical error prevention*. StatPearls [Internet]. Treasure Island (FL): StatPearls Publishing.

Rosaldo, M. Z. (1980). *Knowledge and passion* (Vol. 4). Cambridge: Cambridge University Press.

RosBusinessConsulting. (2020). Russian doctors wrote a letter to Putin in support of neonatologist Sushkevich: https://kaliningrad.rbc.ru/kaliningrad/01/12/2020/5fc64aa89a7947289194f575?from=copy (in Russian).

Rose, N. (1998). *Inventing our selves: Psychology, power, and personhood.* Cambridge: Cambridge University Press.

Rose, N., & Novas, C. (2005). Biological citizenship, in Ong A., Collier S.J. (Eds.), *Global assemblages: Technology, politics, and ethics as anthropological problems* (pp. 439–463). Blackwell.

Rosenberg, C. E. (2002). The tyranny of diagnosis: Specific entities and individual experience. *The Milbank Quarterly*, 80(2), 237–260.

Rosenhan, D. L. (1973). On being sane in insane places. *Science*, 179(4070), 250–258.

Roth, Julius A. (1972). Some contingencies of the moral evaluation and control of Clientele: The case of the hospital emergency service. *American Journal of Sociology* 77(5), 839–856.

Saks, M. (2015). *The professions, state and the market: Medicine in Britain, the United States and Russia.* New York: Routledge.

Salander, P., Bergenheim, T., & Henriksson, R. (1996). The creation of protection and hope in patients with malignant brain tumours. *Social Science & Medicine*, 42(7), 985–996.

Scheer, M. (2012). Are emotions a kind of practice (and is that what makes them have a history)? A Bourdieuian approach to understanding emotion. *History and Theory*, 51(2), 193–220.

Scheper-Hughes, N., & Lock, M. M. (1987). The mindful body: A prolegomenon to future work in medical anthropology. *Medical Anthropology Quarterly*, 1(1), 6–41.

Sergeeva, O. V., & Zinenko Yu. V. Features of conducting checks on reports of crimes related to the provision of medical care. Criminalistics: Yesterday, today, tomorrow. 2021. 19(3). 157–164. (in Russ.). https://doi.org/10.24412/2587-9820-2021-3-157-164.

Shabalov, N. P., & Alexandrovich, Y. S. (2018). Eduard Kuzmich Tsybul'kin the founder of critical and emergency care for children in Saint-Petersburg (the 80th anniversary of his birth). *Pediatr*, 9(5), 131–138. (in Russian).

Sheiman, I., Shishkin, S., and Shevsky, V. (2018). The evolving Semashko model of primary health care: The case of the Russian Federation. *Risk Management and Healthcare Policy*, 11, 209.

Shevchenko, N. (2023). Bureaucratic routes and documentary temporalities of the conscript's questionnaire in a human rights organization. *Anthropological Forum*, 59, 73–102. (in Russian).

Smithson, J. (2000). Using and analysing focus groups: Limitations and possibilities. *International Journal of Social Research Methodology*, 3(2), 103–119.

Solomon, P. (2018). Accusatorial bias in Russian criminal justice, in Kurkchiyan, M., & Kubal, A. (Eds.), *A sociology of justice in Russia* (pp. 170–204). Cambridge University Press. New York: Cambridge University Press.

Speransky, G. N. (1914). Experience of the device and maintenance of a special hospital for infants [Opyt ustrojstva i vedeniya special'noj lechebnicy dlya detej grudnogo vozrasta]. Materials on the study of infancy. Vol. 1 / edited by G. N. Speransky. M.: Treatment center for infants. P. 10–19.] (in Russian).

Star, S. L. (1999). The ethnography of infrastructure. *American Behavioral Scientist*, 43(3), 377–391.

Starodubov, V. I., & Sukhanova, L. P. (2013). New criteria of birth: Medical and demographical outcomes and organizational problems of obstetrics service [Novye kriterii rozhdeniya: mediko-demograficheskie rezul'taty i organizacionnye problemy sluzhby rodovspomozheniya]. Manager Zdravoochranenia ISSN 1811-0185, (12), 21–29. (in Russian).

Strauss, A., Schatzman, L., Ehrlich, D., Bucher, R., & Sabshin, M. (1963). The hospital and its negotiated order, in Freidson E. (Ed.), *The hospital in modern society* (pp. 147–169). London: The Free Press.

Tarasenko, A. (2018). Russian non-profit organisations in service delivery: Neoliberal and statist social policy principles intertwined. *Europe-Asia Studies*, 70(4), 514–530.

Temkina, A. A. (2017). 'Ekonomika doveriya' v platnom segmente rodovspomozheniya: gorodskaya obrazovannaya zhenshchina kak potrebitel' i patsientka ['The Economy of Trust' in the Paied-for Maternity Care: Urban Educated Woman as a Consumer and a Patient], Ekonomicheskaya sotsiologiya [Economic Sociology], 18(3), 14–53.

Temkina, A. A. (2014). Medicalization of reproduction and childbirth: A struggle for control. *Journal of Social Policy Studies*, 12(3), 321–336. (in Russian).

Temkina, A., & Rivkin-Fish, M. (2020). Creating health care consumers: The negotiation of un/official payments, power and trust in Russian maternity care. *Social Theory & Health*, 18, 340–357.

Temkina, A., Litvina, D., & Novkunskaya, A. (2021). Emotional styles in Russian maternity hospitals: Juggling between khamstvo and smiling. *Emotions and Society*, 3(1), 95–113.

Temkina, A., Novkunskaya, A., & Litvina, D. (2022). *Pregnancy and birth in Russia: The struggle for "good care"*. Milton Park: Taylor & Francis.

The law of the Kaliningrad Region issued on November 29, 2023, No. 279 "On the prohibition of inducement to induce artificial termination of pregnancy in the Kaliningrad region", Adopted by the Legislative Assembly of the Kaliningrad region (seventh convocation) on November 22, 2023. Available at: https://www.garant.ru/hotlaw/kaliningrad/1664298/ (access date 09.01.2024) (in Russian).

The Law of the Pskov Oblast "On Prohibition of Inducement of Artificial Termination of Pregnancy in the Pskov Oblast" was adopted by the Pskov Oblast Assembly of Deputies on December 25, 2023. Available at: https://pskov.ru/sites/default/files/documents/2023/2442-oz.pdf (access date 09.01.2024).

Tolstikova, O. M. (2017). Problems of legal regulation of surrogate motherhood in Russia. *Siberian Legal Bulletin*, 1, 83–87. (in Russian).

Torchin, H., Morgan, A. S., & Ancel, P. Y. (2020, June). International comparisons of neurodevelopmental outcomes in infants born very preterm, in *Seminars in fetal and neonatal medicine* (Vol. 25, No. 3, p. 101109). Philadelphia: WB Saunders.

Turner, V. W. (1969). *The ritual process: Structure and anti-structure*. New York: Routledge. Harmonds-worth.

Ugarova, A. (2018). Strong drug: Illigal prescription of drug painkillers and legal cases against physicians, *ES Forum Bulletin*, 2(58), 6–12. (In Russian).

Uspensky, V. P. (1911). Moscow. Brief sketch of development and modern state of city medical and sanitary organization [Kratkij ocherk razvitiya i sovremennogo sostoyaniya gorodskoj vrachebno-sanitarnoj organizacii]. Edition of the City Administration. Moscow: Gorodskaya Tipografiya (p. 131). (in Russian).

Van Nistelrooij, I., Visse, M., Spekkink, A., & de Lange, J. (2017). How shared is shared decision-making? A care-ethical view on the role of partner and family. *Journal of Medical Ethics*, 43(9), 637–644.

Vigotsky, L. S. (1939). Thought and speech. *Psychiatry*, 2(1), 29–54.

Volodin, N. N. (2020). Open letter regarding the Elina Sushkevich case. *Obstetrics, Gynecology and Reproduction*, 14(6), 704–709.

Volodin, N. N., Sukhikh, G. T., Baibarina, E. N., & Ryumina, I. I. (2008). *Basic care for the newborn-international experience* [Bazovaya pomoshch' novorozhdyonnomu — mezhdunarodnyj opyt]. Geotar-Media. (in Russian).

Wamsiedel, M. (2016). Lay values, organizational concerns, and the handling of 'social cases' in Romanian emergency departments. *Transylvanian Review*, 25(1), 61–76.

Wamsiedel, M. (2020). Credibility work and moral evaluation at the ED. *Social Science & Medicine*, 248(112845), 1–8.

Wamsiedel, M. (2023). The moral evaluation of emergency department patients: An ethnography of triage work in Romania. Lanham: Rowman & Littlefield.

World Health Organization. (2010). *International statistical classification of diseases and related health problems*. 10th revision, edition 2010 (ICD-10). World Health Organization.

Zaerko, O. A. (2017). On the shelter establishment for premature infants in St. Petersburg [K voprosu ob osnovanii v Sankt-Peterburge priyuta dlya nedonoshennyh detej]. Scientific Notes of Petrozavodsk State University, (7 (168)), 30–35. (in Russian).

Zola, K. (1972). Medicine as an institution of social control. *Sociological Review*, 20, 487–450.

Index

agency: parents', 158–63, 177, 189; patients', xiii, 43–49, 62, 192; professional, 189
asylum, 2
attention, 51, 55, 68, 74, 79, 81, 88–89
autonomy, xiii–xiv, 129

baby talk, 52, 79–81, 125, 194
birth criteria, 18–19
body, 76, 119, 123, 125, 132, 144, 189–90; bureaucratic, 130; paper, 130–31, 133, 136–41, 152, 175, 180–86, 189–90; physical, 130, 141, 179, 188; weight, 8, 15, 17–19, 71, 75, 112, 128n1
bureaucracy, 133, 140; bureaucratic, 1, 57–58, 115, 124, 129–42, 147, 156, 159–65, 172, 179, 186, 189–90, 194; paperwork, 103, 138–42, 147, 153, 180

care: high-tech, 21, 151, 153, 177; intensive, 4, 6–10, 13, 16–17, 20–22, 28, 29, 33, 51–59, 62, 65–66, 70, 74–75, 81–86, 96–105, 108, 110, 117, 119, 127, 141, 146, 178–81, 188; maternity, 48, 57; medical, 2, 7, 9, 12, 19–21, 44, 57–58, 66, 72, 84, 131–32, 139, 141, 145, 151, 155, 157, 160, 169–74, 179, 185; neonatal, 1, 6–7, 18–20, 22–23, 49, 52, 67, 71, 75–77, 88, 125, 127, 129–36, 141–45, 149–53, 161–62, 169, 186, 189; for newborn(s), 1, 4, 6, 14–16, 19, 22, 176, 181; object(s) of, 103, 110; obstetric, 5, 20–21, 141, 159, 160; palliative, 23, 127, 181; for pregnant women, 6, 18; primary, 99, 112, 113, 125, 126; sectors of, 70, 72, 78, 81, 87, 92, 107, 112, 115, 122, 126–27, 137, 166, 191; specialized, 7–8, 16, 21, 155; system of, 1, 2, 4, 19–23, 144, 151, 157, 166, 183–86, 189
children, 2–4, 21, 52, 58, 60, 65–66, 72, 75–77, 81–87, 101–3, 121, 177; (with) asphyxia, 9, 84, 124; difficult, 73, 107, 155; with disabilities, 29, 31, 65, 86, 195; doctor's. *See* medical; doubtful, 71, 73, 84; ethnic. *See* foreigner; with extremely low body weight, 14–17, 19, 71, 75; foetus, 9, 38, 54, 62, 75, 128n1, 194; foreigner, 54, 58, 71–72; healthy, 83, 84, 142; incomprehensible. *See* doubtful; late child, 54, 59, 62; medical, 54, 72, 85, 95; palliative, 82, 127; with pathology, 22, 72, 74–75, 77, 194–95; pig in a poke, 73–75,

86, 125; premature, 2–5, 7–10, 14–20, 31, 65–66, 75, 81, 103, 124–25, 172, 195; (un)stable, 75, 81–82, 194; unpromising, 72, 76, 82–83, 127; urgent, 81, 125; without documents, 54, 57–58, 71. *See also* foreigner
citizenship, 57, 72, 115, 151, 181–85; non-Russian, 115, 151, 181, 186, 190
clinics, 2, 6–7, 15, 21–22, 48, 161; private, 21–22, 48–49; private maternity, 28, 59, 151, 158, 161
communication, 11–12, 28–30, 44–46, 48–51, 69, 79, 81, 83, 90, 97–99, 107, 113, 115; communicative intention, 44; communicative registries, 43, 45, 150; communicative work, 94, 97, 114; informal, 58; medical, 46, 59, 101; non-verbal, 68; with parents, 93–94, 97–99, 102, 103, 106, 124, 126; with patients, 60, 69, 79–81, 83, 93, 129; professional, 51, 55, 59–60, 94, 96, 190–91
competition, 15–17, 142, 153; professional, 17
complications, 20–23, 162
coping strategies, xiii, 70
COVID-19 pandemic, xiii, 41, 178, 197
crying, 46–47, 79, 96, 116, 196

death, 12, 17, 31, 62, 67, 72, 77, 86, 171, 176, 187; probability of, 127, 162, 174; reporting the, 100–101

emotions, 30, 39, 66–69, 83, 89, 96–98, 104, 109, 113, 115–18, 125–27; embodied, 68; emotional burnout, 70, 119, 134; emotional fatigue, 38, 67, 90, 115–19; emotional work, 73, 97, 101, 114; expressing emotions, 69, 70; manifestation of, 66, 96, 116, 191; performance of, 69, 79; restraining, 113, 116, 126
entity, 74, 133, 136, 183, 184, 186, 189; bureaucratic, 133, 135, 137, 179; economic, 130; legal, 131, 177, 179; political, 130, 162, 164, 177; social, 188
expertise, 3, 12, 33, 39, 141–42, 167, 169, 171, 174

family, 55, 86–88, 107, 119, 132, 151, 190; 'family births', 59. *See also* parents

gender, 31, 32, 38, 43–44, 47–51, 80, 95, 132
gestational age, 8, 19, 163
Goffman, Erving, 12, 62, 69, 94, 129, 132
gynaecological departments, 8, 16, 19

healthcare, 48, 151, 160–61, 170; managers, 16, 130, 153, 163, 188; organizers. *See* managers; policies, 160; public, 49; Russian, 147, 173, 187; system, 12, 129, 160
history, 1–5, 15, 26, 124, 179, 189; medical, 71, 125, 130, 133, 151, 155; patient, 75, 87, 153; patient without, 71, 74; the region of, 6
Hochschild, Arlie, 69–70, 104
hospital, 5, 8–9, 13, 150, 152–58, 191; children's, 2, 6–7, 14–17, 21–23, 52, 74, 126, 145, 169, 180; city, 10, 28, 145; hospitalization, 20–21, 43, 103, 129–31, 138, 142, 146, 153, 157–58, 182–85, 190; maternity, 3–7, 10–11, 13–14, 20–22, 23n2, 28, 50, 53, 60, 71–74, 77, 86, 92–100, 126, 142, 145, 149, 155, 161; multidisciplinary, x, 21–23, 59; paediatric. *See* children's; private, 21–22, 28, 48–49, 59, 151, 158
human resources, 103, 105, 149–50

infant mortality, 3–4, 15, 135, 160–63, 174
informal, 50, 58, 114, 159, 167, 183; control, 12; hierarchy, 107–8; rules, 132–35, 141, 158, 170

infrastructure, 7, 119, 130, 141–49, 160, 178–79, 183, 189
inpatient, x, 5, 10, 23, 59, 62, 81, 180
institution, 1–7, 16, 20–22, 44–46, 69–70, 92, 121–22, 145, 149, 153, 162; closed, xiv, 12, 33; institutional context, 35, 68, 96, 127, 170, 188; institutionalization, 1, 4, 31, 43; quasi-total, 12
insurance: companies, 135, 152, 166; funds, 58, 151; mandatory health insurance (MHI), 21, 152; policy, 57–58, 134–35, 158, 185
intensive care, 6, 62, 66, 74, 84, 86, 98–99, 102, 146, 178–81; beds, 7, 17, 22; neonatal intensive care unit (NICU), 6–7, 13, 20; unit, 6–10, 13, 16–17, 33, 52–53, 82, 84, 97, 119
interaction: interactionist perspective, 43–45, 69; with parents, 62, 70, 72, 85–92, 97, 100, 102; with patients, 43, 45–49, 51–53, 70, 78–81, 129, 190; between professionals, 12, 27, 69–70, 107–9, 113–14, 126
IVF. *See* in vitro fertilization (IVF)

knowledge, 1, 12, 62, 165, 192; medical, 6, 26; professional, 60, 71, 141, 164

labelling theory, 43, 45–46
labels, 38, 43–48, 53–62, 71, 85, 128n1, 170, 179, 187, 190
law enforcement, 129, 131, 135, 170, 173–76; agencies, 166; practices, 129, 163, 169–70
legal: context, 18, 131, 163, 170, 177; environment, 169–71, 173; framework, 22; norms, 170; risks, 12, 131; status of a newborn, 18, 129, 184–85
logics: bureaucratic, 172, 186; managerial, 129, 169; market, 129, 154–55; professional, 129, 141, 157–58, 165, 186; of regulation, 129, 160, 162–63

material resources, 130, 141, 143, 147, 169
medical: categories, 43, 45; communication, 33, 59, 101, 130, 133; errors, 12, 124, 194; ethics, 83, 118, 163, 170; gaze, ix, xii, 13, 188; hierarchy, 110; knowledge, 26, 192; labels, 38, 48, 53, 56, 60, 62, 85; organizations, 11–12, 130, 133, 140–41, 151–52, 166
medicalization, 6, 20, 43–46, 61–62, 72, 132, 141, 190, 192, 195
MHI. *See* mandatory health insurance (MHI)
moral: career, 62; neutrality, 62; resources, 76, 100, 194–95; responsibility, 77, 124

negotiated order, 135, 165
NICU. *See* neonatal intensive care unit (NICU)
norms: cultural, 81, 126, 186–87; ethical, 39; informal, 170; legal, 169–70, 186; normative scenario, 96, 98; organizational, 36; social, 44, 188
NRAC. *See* Resuscitation and Advisory Centre (NRAC)

objectification, xii, 43, 45
obstetrics and gynecology, ix, 3–6, 21, 110, 136, 160, 171

palliative: care centres, 23; patients, 82–83, 127; services, 22; status, 86, 102, 194
Parsons, Talcott, ix, 43–44, 86
participant observation, 40–41, 68, 209
patient, ix–x, 1, 12, 22, 35, 43–44, 47–49, 53, 62, 124–27, 181–90; career, 129, 132; chronic, 82; death of a, 17, 31, 72, 77, 86, 100–101, 127, 162, 174–76, 190; extended, 33, 43, 62, 72, 86, 89, 126, 135, 156, 190;

obstetric, 19; palliative. *See* palliative patients; paper, 133, 135; relatives, 12, 59–60, 89, 100, 104, 106, 116, 123, 187–88, 192; without a personal biography, 35, 71, 74–75. *See also* patient without history
performance indicators, xiii, 135, 160–61
phenomenological experience, 68
professional: autonomy, 129; burnout, 121, 127. *See also* emotional burnout; communication, 55, 96, 190; community, 4, 15, 19, 54, 76, 130, 156, 163–66, 172; hierarchy, 167; identity, 87, 92, 119–20, 126, 191; networks, 60; practices, 19, 144, 159, 169, 175; professionalism, 66, 71, 74, 78, 82, 91, 142, 163–65, 170, 179, 195. *See also* logics professional; professionalization of emotions, 117–18; responsibility, 75, 101; socialization, 30, 50; standards, 18, 35
pronatalism, 160–61

quality of life, 18

RAC. *See* resuscitation and advisory centre (RAC)
research position, xi, 25–27, 32–34, 40, 189, 191
resuscitation, 12, 16, 18, 59, 83, 86, 141, 153, 176, 179; and Advisory Centre (RAC), 7, 22, 49, 93, 150; mandatory resuscitation, 18, 163, 176; team, 73, 93, 113, 145, 149; unit, 6, 20, 121, 126
risk: of complications, 20, 162; legal, 12, 45, 124, 131, 174–76; reputational, 33; of unfavorable outcomes, 10, 35; women at, 6
role: gender, 91; of the researchers, 25, 29; sick, 43–44; social, 43, 81
rules: bureaucratic, 129, 139, 142, 163; of emotional display, 69; formal, 129, 132, 170, 179, 184, 188; of interaction, 44, 48; medical, 1, 83

Scheer, Monique, 68–69, 73, 79, 126
sensitive issues, 36–37, 39
social: categories. *See* labels; sociocultural contexts, 40, 45, 141; status, 5, 31, 43, 48, 54, 103, 130, 132, 140, 177, 186
state control, 160
statistics, 12, 19, 77, 172
stereotypes, 47, 80, 125, 190
surgical pathology, 6, 10, 15, 74

team: research, 28, 32–34, 195, 197; resuscitation, 73; teamwork, 107–10; transport, 8, 29, 73, 92–94, 97, 113–14, 128n3. *See also* resuscitation and advisory centre
technologies, 10, 14–15, 124, 179, 183–84, 194
trajectories: patient, 46, 62–63, 71, 129–31, 157, 182, 185, 190; treatment, 44, 54, 60, 169, 184, 187
triage, x, 62, 71, 76
trust, 13, 29, 66, 106, 110

vernacular instruments, 146
vital functions, 22, 151
in vitro fertilization (IVF), 54–55, 59, 62, 126, 195

wellbeing, 72, 96
WHO. *See* World Health Organization (WHO)
work routine, 43, 67–69
World Health Organization (WHO), 18

About the Authors

Anastasia Novkunskaya is a sociologist and associate professor of qualitative health research at the Institute for Interdisciplinary Health Research at the European University at Saint Petersburg. She received her PhD in Social Sciences at the University of Helsinki in 2020. Anastasia's key research fields are the sociology of health and medicine, the sociology of professions and qualitative methodology. Her work in these areas has been published in multiple journals, including *Scientific Reports, Health: An Interdisciplinary Journal for the Social Study of Health, Illness and Medicine*, *Emotions and Society*, *Laboratorium: Russian Review of Social Research* and *Europe-Asia Studies*. She is also co-author of *Pregnancy and Birth in Russia: The Struggle for 'Good Care'* published in 2022.

Artemiy Minakov is a research fellow at the Institute for Interdisciplinary Health Research at the European University at Saint Petersburg, an analyst of social research in medicine, practising doctor at the Neonatal Intensive Care Unit and the Head of the Resuscitation-Advisory Centre. His main fields of research interest are intensive care in neonatology and interprofessional communication. In addition, Artemiy used to be a psychiatry resident, with his main area of interest being in endogenous psychoses and social adaptation through religious and traditional beliefs.

Anna Klepikova holds a PhD in cultural anthropology. She has worked on several projects in the fields of disability studies and medical anthropology. Her research has focused on institutions for people with multiple disabilities, family care for disabled children and adults, organisation and experiences of palliative care, complementary and alternative medicine, and religious healing. She teaches courses in medical anthropology and fieldwork methods. She has published a book, *I Must Be a Fool: Anthropological Novel* (in Russian), dedicated to the state-run institutions for people with disabilities and contrasting ideologies and practices of public care to those offered by grassroot organizations. The English translation of the book will be published in 2024–2025.

www.ingramcontent.com/pod-product-compliance
Lightning Source LLC
LaVergne TN
LVHW091529200926
848483LV00002B/338
9781666937404